J. BUKOWSKI

The Mind Has Mountains

The Mind Has Mountains

Reflections on Society and Psychiatry

Paul R. McHugh, M.D.

The Johns Hopkins University Press

Baltimore

© 2006 The Johns Hopkins University Press
All rights reserved. Published 2006
Printed in the United States of America on acid-free paper
9 8 7 6 5 4 3 2 1

The Johns Hopkins University Press
2715 North Charles Street
Baltimore, Maryland 21218-4363
www.press.jhu.edu

Library of Congress Cataloging-in-Publication Data
McHugh, Paul R. (Paul Rodney), 1931–
    The mind has mountains : reflections on society and psychiatry / Paul R. McHugh.
        p. ; cm.
    Includes bibliographical references.
    ISBN 0-8018-8249-4 (hardcover : alk. paper)
    1. Psychiatry. 2. Psychiatry—Philosophy.
    [DNLM: 1. Psychiatry—Collected Works. 2. Mental Disorders—Collected Works.
3. Philosophy, Medical—Collected Works. 4. Psychological Theory—Collected Works.
WM 100 M478m 2005] I. Title.
    RC458.M33 2005
    616.89—dc22   2005007793

A catalog record for this book is available from the British Library.

The last two printed pages of this book are an extension of this copyright page.

Once more, for Jean

O the mind, mind has mountains; cliffs of fall

Frightful, sheer, no-man-fathomed. Hold them cheap

May who ne'er hung there.

—Gerard Manley Hopkins

CONTENTS

PREFACE

The essays in this book were in one way or another prompted by disbelief in many claims and opinions expressed by psychiatrists and psychologists of my generation. I sensed a detrimental collaboration developing between some psychiatric teachers and champions of the contemporary culture which was depriving the discipline of coherence and encouraging the worst features of the times. Psychiatrists made claims that were not true, pressed for attitudes and behaviors that were destructive, and held beliefs about human mental life that were incredible. All these ideas were both transmitted to and reciprocally evoked by a civilization already confused about matters of truth and morals. In writing these essays I began to object to this state of affairs and to offer ways of thinking about mental life and mental illness that would offer more coherent and productive lines of inference for both the discipline and the social order.

Each of the essays tried to challenge or amend some egregious thought or practice in psychiatry. Some were prompted by an episode in the news in which psychiatric opinions were misemployed, usually because of an extension of a school of thought beyond its limits. Others are responses to books offering directions for patient care and treatment that seemed mischievous. Among these essays the reader can find one of the first salvos fired in the "memory wars" against claims about multiple personality disorder and repressed memory of sexual abuse. But also included are criticisms of physician-assisted suicide, the overprescription of psychotropic medications, the overdiagnosis and inappropriate treatment of post-traumatic stress disorder, and even the cultural ethos expressed in the weirdly <u>bowdlerized</u> forms of the Hippocratic Oath taken by contemporary medical school graduates.

Most of the essays speak for themselves. Let me draw out two themes that are implicit in all of them. The first theme is my instinctive antipathy toward what can be called the "Gnostic" presumptions that often emerge in psychiatric discourse, views, and even practices. Here fall the various assumptions that psychiatrists know deep secrets, having been initiated into them by a unique kind of education and experience. These secrets tend to turn on matters sexual, rest upon unconscious drives and conflicts, and usually carry both a criticism of traditional morals and a sense that psychotherapy can offer a salvational conversion from the dominance of a depriving, puritanical culture. I think most of these ideas are wrongheaded and have in the past generated strange routines and teachings. This theme is exemplified best in the essay "What's the Story?" which tries to capture among other experiences the antics of the teachers of psychiatry I encountered as a student at Harvard Medical School.

The second theme in the essays concerns another (and perhaps now the more prominent) element of contemporary psychiatry giving root support to misdirections, an element that has less of an insidious feature than the Gnostic presumptions. Psychotherapists have a natural tendency to give themselves over to the softer virtues of kindness, gentleness, and soothing support (often saluted as "nonjudgmental") at the expense of the sterner virtues of truth, responsibility, and justice. As Shirley Robin Letwin pointed out in her brilliant assessment, *The Anatomy of Thatcherism* (1992), the sterner—or, as she referred to them, "vigorous"—virtues are not incompatible with kindness and support. One can be truthful and kind, just and gentle, but it is often a matter of emphasis. The proper balance is difficult to strike when we psychotherapists must make a hard truth palatable for patients whose behaviors are getting them into trouble even as they are set on indulging them. Then we are coaxed to permit the softer virtues of kindness, understanding, and support to move forward at the expense of honesty and prudence, to the ultimate detriment of the patient and the public's attitude toward the discipline itself. Perhaps the best example here is the fad for sexual reassignment surgery that has so disrupted coherent thought over human nature in the recent years, discussed here in the essay "Psychiatric Misadventures" and followed up in the essay "Surgical Sex."

To avoid an unrelenting stance of criticism against psychiatry that provides no solutions to its problems or general response to its predicament, the book concludes with essays that describe the systematic ways of thinking about psychiatric disorders taught at the Johns Hopkins University School of Medicine and how these ways work for the benefit of patients and support the discipline generally. This section also encompasses a discussion of the formative ideas psychiatry gained from Karl Jaspers; a consideration of the inspiration all medical disciplines take from William Osler, the founding professor of the Department of Medicine at Johns Hopkins; and a discussion of the mind/brain problem as a major source of some discord in this field. I close with a review of the history of the "memory wars" and how the Harvard psychologist Richard J. McNally, in writing the book *Remembering Trauma* (2003), resolved this confusion in psychiatric thought and practice.

In the Department of Psychiatry at Johns Hopkins we hold and promote the view that psychiatry—as it struggles to find its proper place in contemporary medicine—must opt for an intellectual stance of constructive realism, linking its observations and its explanations to what can be seen to exist. Only this stance will provide it with both the ability to engage in an honest, open dialogue with the patients it intends to help and the proper authority to advance public understanding of the mentally ill and the services needed for their care. This book—along with one coauthored with Phillip R. Slavney, *The Perspectives of Psychiatry* (1998), describing in more detail my concepts for the structure of this clinical discipline—represents efforts to develop that stance and to cultivate the discourse that will lead to these happy outcomes.

ACKNOWLEDGMENTS

All of these essays at root emerged from encouragement I received from two men. Dr. Richard Starr Ross, the dean of the Johns Hopkins School of Medicine (and arguably the finest dean at Hopkins since William Welch), was the first to insist that I strive to explain to the public the implications of our department's conceptions on psychiatry. Joseph Epstein, the editor of the *American Scholar* (and arguably the finest essayist writing in English today), provided me the first opportunities to publish my thoughts and in the process taught me how to translate my opinions from the professional jargon that comes easily to a doctor into coherent argument. I owe a great debt of gratitude to the rousing advice of Dean Ross and the gracious instructions of Joseph Epstein.

Neal Kozodoy, editor of *Commentary*, Jane Nevins, of *Dana-Cerebrum*, Father Richard Neuhaus, of *First Things*, Eugene Brody, of the *Journal of Nervous and Mental Disease*, Barbara Culliton, of *Nature Medicine*, Gregory Curfman, of the *New England Journal of Medicine*, and Joseph Bottum and Claudia Winkler, of the *Weekly Standard* all prompted me to venture forth on one or another of these essays and were willing to open the pages of their distinguished journals to my ideas. Their wise editorial counsel greatly helped me shape each product.

Although the opinions expressed here are my responsibility, I have over the years been enriched by thoughts and concepts received from critical conversations and correspondence with many friends and colleagues: Patrick Barta, David Blass, Joseph Brady, Jason Brandt, Michael Clark, Sandra Costich, Frederick Crews, Raymond DePaulo, William Eaton, David Edwin, Marshal Folstein, Susan Folstein, Jerome Frank, Pamela Freyd, Michael Gazzaniga, Leon Kass, Robert Leavitt, S.S., Harold Lief, Elizabeth Loftus, Constantine Lyketsos, Francis McMahon, Richard McNally, Jon Meyer, Timothy Moran, Gerald Nestadt, Martin Orne, Michael Pakenham, Godfrey Pearlson, Peter Rabins, William Reiner, Alan Romanoski, Michael

Sandel, Patricia Santora, Phillip Slavney, Owsei Temkin, Glenn Treis-
man, and Tom Wolfe.

The editors at the Johns Hopkins University Press have been
superb collaborators. Grace Carino worked meticulously over each
essay and Trevor Lipscombe enhanced the heft and integrity of
the whole enterprise with valuable suggestions and illuminating
thoughts. My secretary Barbara Cross was ever helpful and diligent in
preparing the manuscripts.

Finally, I was sustained by Jean Barlow McHugh, who not only
encouraged these efforts but demonstrated an incredible aptitude for
drawing corrective attention to some muddle (sometimes several)
that initially flawed each essay. The dedication of this volume can
represent but a modest tribute to the many and manifold ways she
has enriched my life and discernments for over forty-six years.

Part I

THE BEGINNING

One learns early that teaching psychiatry resembles practicing it. You must knock bad ideas out of heads before you can start putting good ones in. You also learn—from both experiences—that bad ideas have a strong grip on people.

The essays in this part of the book represent my first attempts at raising public attention to some of the bad ideas floating around in psychiatry at the time. There were several of them, as you can see. Some of them—such as those of Thomas Szasz—might best be described as half-truths: in Szasz's case, for instance, he was calling attention to some overconfidence in the discipline but was offering no coherent program for correcting it. Others were clear misdirections of thought and action already producing victims who needed to be identified. Here I include the sex-change surgeries that were in vogue and also the emerging concepts of repressed memories of sex abuse and multiple personalities that did great damage to families and to the standing of psychotherapy in America.

I often wondered where these ideas got such energy and—as I learned as I began to oppose them—such staying power given that they so obviously seemed to be forms of enmity to both the moral hostility antagonism *imperatives and intellect's commands on doctors to "do no harm." I concluded that psychiatrists were vulnerable to a "romantic" impulse to believe in things so mysterious in the human mind that only initiates to the secrets could appreciate them.*

Many psychiatrists hungered to discern the hidden forces of "power" in our world that exploited human mental weaknesses and, these psychiatrists were convinced, were producing many victims. Other psychiatrists were simply intent on belonging to the "knowers" (the "gnosteosie") of their times who discerned a "truer" reality behind perceptible things from whence ineluctable laws of mental life and

1

nature emerged. These latter seemed the psychiatric counterparts of the twentieth century's political romancers who promoted communism and fascism through attitudes of utopianism and intolerance that the scientific enlightenment often carried.

These psychiatric intentions—hurtful not through malice but through hubris—represented vulnerabilities of my discipline and produced the ideas and practices that I wanted to purge. Here are my attempts to describe them to a discerning public—and to any in my profession interested in discussing them—so as, I hoped, to build a resistance to them and to the "romantic" impulse that generated them.

Psychiatric Misadventures

Psychiatry is a rudimentary medical art. It lacks easy access to proof of its proposals even as it deals with disorders of the most complex features of human life—mind and behavior. Yet, probably because of the earlier examples of Freud and Jung, a belief persists that psychiatrists are entitled to special privileges—that they know the secret of human nature—and thus can venture beyond their clinic-based competencies to instruct on nonmedical matters: interpreting literature, counseling the electorate, prescribing for the millennium.

At the Johns Hopkins University, my better days are spent teaching psychiatry to residents and medical students. As I attempt to make clear to them what psychiatrists actually do know and how they know it, I am often aware that I am drawing them back from trendy thought, redirecting them from salvationist aspirations toward the *Theme* traditional concerns of psychiatry, which is about the differentiation, understanding, and treatment of the mentally ill.

Part of my justification for curbing my students' expansive impulses is that they have enough to learn, and several things to unlearn, about patients. Such sciences as epidemiology, genetics, and neuropharmacology, which support and surround psychiatry today, are bringing new power to our practice, just as science did for internal medicine and surgery earlier in this century. Only those physicians with critical capacities—who see the conceptual structure of this discipline and can distinguish valid from invalid opinions—will be competent to make use of these new scientific concepts and technologies in productive ways. I want my students to number among those who will transform psychiatry in the future.

But my other justification for corralling their enthusiasms is the sense that the intermingling of psychiatry with contemporary culture is excessive and injures both parties. During the thirty years of my professional experience, I have witnessed the power of cultural fashion to leave psychiatric thought and practice off in false, even disastrous, directions. I have become familiar with how these fashions and their consequences caused psychiatry to lose its moorings. Roughly

3

every ten years, from the mid-1960s on, psychiatric practice has condoned some bizarre misdirection, proving how all too often the discipline has been the captive of the culture.

Each misdirection was the consequence of one of three common medical mistakes—oversimplification, misplaced emphasis, or pure invention. Psychiatry may be more vulnerable to such errors than other clinical endeavors, given its lack of checks and correctives, such as the autopsies and laboratory tests that protect other medical specialties. But for each error, cultural fashion provided the inclination and the impetus. When caught up by the social suppositions of their time, psychiatrists can do much harm.

The most conspicuous misdirection of psychiatric practice—the precipitate dismissal of patients with severe, chronic mental disorders such as schizophrenia from psychiatric hospitals—certainly required a vastly oversimplified view of mental illness. These actions were defended as efforts to bring "freedom" to these people, sounding a typical 1960s theme, as though it were not their illnesses but society that deprived them of freedom in the first place.

There were several collaborators in this sad enterprise—prominent among them the state governments looking for release from the traditional but heavy fiscal burden of housing the mentally ill. Crucial to the process were the fashionable opinions of the time about society's institutions and, specifically, the oversimplified opinions about schizophrenia and other mental illnesses generated by the so-called antipsychiatrists: Thomas Szasz, R. D. Laing, Erving Goffman, Michel Foucault, and the rest. These men provided an acid commentary on psychiatric thought and practice, which in turn eroded confidence in the spirit of psychiatric concern for the mentally ill that had previously generated, and regularly regenerated, advocacy on the part of mainstream psychiatry for their welfare. This traditional concern had lasted for more than 120 years in America, or ever since the 1840s crusades led by Dorothea Dix to provide professional services and humane conditions for the mentally ill.

The "antipsychiatry" school depicted mental institutions as medically useless, self-serving institutions run for the management and quite unnecessary for patients. These commentators scorned social attitudes about the mentally ill and the contemporary psychiatric practice, but not one of them described the impairments of mind in patients with schizophrenia, manic-depressive illness, or mental retardation or senility. Data about these impairments were what Dix and an enlightened public came to emphasize when founding psychiatrically supervised, state-supported hospitals. These hospitals rescued the mentally ill from destitution, jails, and the mean streets of cities.

Description of the mental problems of psychiatric patients was not the style of the popular 1960s commentators. They were more interested in painting a picture of their own devising that would provoke first suspicion and then disdain for contemporary psychiatric practices and did so not by producing new standards or reforming specific practices but by ridiculing, and caricaturing efforts of the institutions and people at hand just as fashion directed. The power of their scorn was surprising and had amazing results, leading many to believe that it was the institutions that provoked the patients' illnesses rather than the illnesses that called out for shelter and treatment.

Here, from Szasz's book *Schizophrenia: The Sacred Symbol of Psychiatry* (1976), is a typical comment:

> The sense in which I mean that Psychiatry creates schizophrenia is readily illustrated by the analogy between institutional psychiatry and involuntary servitude. If there is no slavery there can be no slaves. . . . Similarly if there is no psychiatry there can be no schizophrenics. In other words, the identity of an individual as a schizophrenic depends on the existence of the social system of [institutional] psychiatry.

The only reply to such commentary is to know the patients for what they are—in schizophrenia, people disabled by delusions, hallucinations, and disruptions of thinking capacities—and to reject an approach that would trivialize their impairments and deny them their frequent need for hospital care.

On one occasion in the early 1970s, when I was working at Cornell University Medical Center in New York, a friend and senior member of the biochemistry faculty called me about a medical student who was balking over a term paper because his career plan was to become a champion of the "psychiatrically oppressed." Biochemistry term papers seemed "irrelevant." Could I offer him a project with psychiatric patients that might be developed into a term paper satisfying the requirements of her department? "He's a neat guy," she said, "but he is stubborn about this and full of views about contemporary psychiatry."

"Send him over," I said, but I awaited his arrival with some apprehension. I needn't have feared the encounter because, in contrast to many other students of those times, he was not looking for a fight. "It's just that I know what I want to do—understand the people who are isolated by the label schizophrenia—and help them achieve what they want in life. I've written enough irrelevant papers in my life," he said. He had graduated summa cum laude from Princeton, with a concentration in philosophy, so he certainly had placed a large number of words on paper.

"Have you ever seen anyone with schizophrenia?" I asked.

"Not in the flesh," he said, "but I think I know what you do with them."

"Well," I replied, "I will be glad to have you see one, and let you tell me how to appreciate his choice of an eccentric way of life that he could be released to express."

I had plenty of patients under my care at the time and chose one who was the same age as the student but who had a severe disruption in his thought processes. Even to talk with him was a distressing experience because few of his thoughts were connected and all of them were vaguely tied to delusional beliefs about the world, his family, and our society. He wasn't aggressive or in any way threatening. He was just bewilderingly incoherent. I left the student with the patient, promising to return in half an hour to learn what he thought.

On my return, I found the student subdued. I started, in a slightly teasing way, to ask where he suggested I might send the patient to start his new life—but was quickly cut off by the student, who, finding his voice, said, "That was nothing like what I expected and nothing like what I've read about. Obviously you can't send this poor fellow out of the hospital. Please tell me how you're treating him."

With this evidence confirming my colleague's judgment of the student's basic good nature in what, after all, had been a heartfelt, if inexperienced, opinion, we went on to talk about the impairments and disabilities of patients with serious mental illnesses, their partial responses to combinations of medication and psychological management, and, finally, the meretricious ideas about their treatment that had been promulgated by contemporary fashion and the antipsychiatry critics without making an effort to examine patients.

The student wrote his biochemistry paper on emerging concepts of the neurochemistry of mental disorders. He buckled down in medical school, and he came, after graduation, to join me as a resident psychiatrist and eventually proved to be one of the best doctors I ever taught. We had overcome something together—all out of going to see a patient, recognizing his burdens, and avoiding assumptions about what fashion said we should find.

A saving grace for any medical theory or practice—the thing that spares it *perpetual* thralldom to the gusty winds of fashion—is the patients. They are real, they are around, and a knowledge of their distressing symptoms guards against oversimplification.

The claim that schizophrenic patients are in any sense living an alternative "lifestyle" that our institutions were inhibiting was of course fatuous. It is now obvious to every citizen of our cities that these patients have impaired capacities to comprehend the world and that they need protection and serious active treatment. Without such help, they drift back to precisely the place Dorothea Dix found them 150 years ago. [margin: *cumphrenlly stupid or inane*]

From the faddish idea of institutions as essentially oppressive emerged a nuance that became more dominant as the 1970s progressed. This was that social custom was itself oppressive. In fact, according to this view, all standards by which behaviors are judged are simply matters of opinion—and emotional opinions at that, likely to be enforced but never justified. In the 1970s, this antinomian idea fueled several psychiatric misdirections. [margin: *faith not moral law*]

A challenge to standards can affect at least the discourse in a psychiatric clinic, if not the practice. These challenges are expressed in such slogans as "Do your own thing," "Whose life is it anyway?" "Be sure to get your own," or Joseph Campbell's "Follow your bliss." All these slogans are familiar to psychiatrists trying to redirect confused, depressed, and often self-belittling patients. Such is their pervasiveness in the culture that they may even divert psychiatrists into misplaced emphases in their understanding of patients.

This interrelationship of cultural antinomianism and a psychiatric misplaced emphasis is seen at its grimmest in the practice known as sex-reassignment surgery. I happen to know about this because Johns Hopkins was one of the places in the United States where this practice was given its start. It was part of my intention, when I arrived in Baltimore in 1975, to help end it.

Not uncommonly, a person comes to the clinic and says something like, "As long as I can remember, I've thought I was in the wrong body. True, I've married and had a couple of kids, and I've had a number of homosexual encounters, but always, in the back and now more often in the front of my mind, there's this idea that actually I'm more a woman than a man."

When we ask what he has done about this, the man often says, "I've tried dressing like a woman and feel quite comfortable. I've even made myself up and gone out in public. I can get away with it because it's all so natural to me. I'm here because all this male equipment is disgusting to me. I want medical help to change my body: hormone treatments, silicone implants, surgical amputation of my genitalia, and the construction of a vagina. Will you do it?"

The patient claims it is a torture for him to live as a man, especially now that he has read in the newspapers about the possibility of switching surgically to womanhood. Upon examination it is not difficult to identify other mental and personality difficulties in him, but he is primarily disquieted because of his intrusive thoughts that his sex is not a settled issue in his life.

Experts say that "gender identity," a sense of one's own maleness or femaleness, is complicated. They believe that it will emerge through the steplike features of most complex developmental processes in which nature and nurture combine. They venture that, although their research on those born with genital and hormonal abnormalities may not apply to a person with normal bodily structures, something must have gone wrong in this patient's early and formative life to cause him to feel as he does. Why not help him look more like what he says he feels? Our surgeons can do it. What the hell!

The skills of our plastic surgeons, particularly on the genitourinary system, are impressive. They were obtained, however, not to treat the gender identity problem but to repair congenital defects, injuries, and the effects of destructive diseases such as cancer in this region of the body.

That you can get something done doesn't always mean that you should do it. In sex-reassignment cases, there are so many problems right at the start. The patient's claim that this has been a lifelong problem is seldom checked with others who have known him since childhood. It seems so intrusive and untrusting to discuss the problem with others, even though they might provide a better gauge of the seriousness of the problem, how it emerged, its fluctuations of intensity over time, and its connection with other experiences. When you discuss what the patient means by "feeling like a woman," you often get a sex stereotype in return—something that female physicians note immediately is a male caricature of women's attitudes and interests. One of our patients, for example, said that, as a woman, he would be more "invested with being than with doing."

It is not obvious how this patient's feeling that he is a woman trapped in a man's body differs from the feeling of a patient with anorexia nervosa that she is obese despite her emaciated, cachectic state. We don't do liposuction on anorexics. Why amputate the genitals of these poor men? Surely, the fault is in the mind, not the member.

Yet, if you justify augmenting breasts for women who feel underendowed, why not do it and more for the man who wants to be a woman? A plastic surgeon at Johns Hopkins provided the voice of reality for me on this matter based on his practice and his natural awe at the mystery of the body. One day while we were talking about it, he said to me: "Imagine what it's like to get up at dawn and think about spending the day slashing with a knife at perfectly well-formed organs because you psychiatrists do not understand what is the problem here but hope surgery may do the poor wretch some good."

The zeal for this sex-change surgery—perhaps, with the exception of frontal lobotomy, the most radical therapy ever encouraged by twentieth-century psychiatrists—did not derive from critical reasoning or thoughtful assessments. These were so faulty that no one holds them up anymore as standards for launching any therapeutic exercise, let alone one so irretrievable as a sex-change operation. The energy came from the fashions of the seventies that invaded the clinic—if you can do it and he wants it, why not do it? It was all tied up with the spirit of doing your thing, following your bliss, an aesthetic that sees diversity as everything and can accept any idea, including that of permanent sex change, as interesting and that views resistance to such ideas as uptight, if not oppressive.

Moral matters should have some salience here. These include the waste of human resources; the confusions imposed on society when these men/women insist on acceptance, even in athletic competition, with women; the encouragement of the "illusion of technique," which assumes that the body is like a suit of clothes to be hemmed and stitched to style; and, finally, the ghastliness of the mutilated anatomy.

But lay these strong moral objections aside and consider only that this surgical practice has distracted effort from genuine investigations attempting to find out just what has gone wrong for these people—what has, by their testimony, given them years of torment and psychological distress and prompted them to accept these grim and disfiguring surgical procedures.

We need to know how to prevent such sadness, indeed horror. We have to learn how to manage this condition as a mental disorder when we fail to prevent it. If it depends on child rearing, then let's learn about its inner dynamics so that parents can be taught to guide their children properly. If it is an aspect of confusion tied to homosexuality, we need to understand its nature and exactly how to manage it as a manifestation of serious mental disorder among homosexual individuals.

But instead of attempting to learn enough to accomplish these worthy goals, psychiatrists collaborated in an exercise of folly with distressed people during a time when "do your own thing" had something akin to the force of a command. As physicians, psychiatrists, when they give in to this, abandon the role of protecting patients from their symptoms and become little more than technicians working on behalf of a cultural force.

Medical errors of oversimplification and misplaced emphasis usually play themselves out for all to see. But the pure inventions bring out a darker, hateful potential when psychiatric thought goes awry. The invention of entities of mind along with their elaborate description, usually fueled by the energy from some social attitude they amplify, is a recurring event in the history of psychiatry.

Most psychiatric histories choose to describe such invention by detailing its most vivid example—witches. The experience in Salem, Massachusetts, of three hundred years ago is prototypical. Briefly, in 1692, several young women and girls who for some weeks had been secretly listening to tales of spells, voodoo, and illicit cultic practices from a Barbados slave suddenly displayed a set of mystifying mental and behavioral changes. They developed trancelike states, falling on the ground and flailing away, and at night and at prayer, seemingly in great distress and in need of help. The local physician, who witnessed this, was as bewildered as anyone else and eventually made a diagnosis of "bewitchment." "The evil hand is on them," he said and turned them over to the local officials for care.

The clergy and magistrates, regarding the young people as victims and pampering them by showing much attention to their symptoms, assumed that local agents of Satan were at work and, using as grounds the answers to leading questions, indicted several citizens. The accepted proof of guilt was bizarre. The young women spoke of visions of the accused, of sensing their presence at night by pains and torments and of ghostly visitations to their homes, all occurring while the accused were known to be elsewhere. The victims even screeched out in court that they felt pinches and pains provoked by the accused, even while the latter were sitting quietly across the room. Judges believed this "spectral" evidence because it conformed to contemporary thought about the capacities of witches; they dismissed all denials of the accused and promptly executed them.

The whole exercise should have been discredited when, after the executions, there was no change in the distraught behavior of the young women. Instead, more and more citizens were indicted. A prosecution depending on "spectral evidence" was at last seen as capricious—as irrefutable as it was undemonstrable. The trials ceased, and eventually several of the young women admitted that their beliefs had been "delusions" and their accusations false.

The modern diagnosis for these young women is, of course, hysteria, not bewitchment. Psychiatrists use the term _hysteria_ to identify behavioral displays in which physical or mental disorders are imitated. The reasons for the behavior vary with the person displaying the disorder but are derived from that person's more or less unconscious effort to appear more significant to others and to be more entitled to their interest and support. The status of the putatively bewitched in Salem in 1692 brought both attentive concern and the license to indict to young women previously scarcely noticed by the community. The forms of hysterical behavior—whether they be physical activities, such as falling and shaking, or mental phenomena, such as pains, visions, or memories—are shaped by unintended suggestions from others and sustained by the attention of onlookers—especially such onlookers as doctors who are socially empowered to assign, by affixing a diagnosis, the status of "patient" to a person. Whenever these diagnosticians mistake hysteria for what it is attempting to imitate—either misidentifying it as a physical illness or inventing some psychological explanation such as bewitchment—then the behavioral display will continue, expand, and, in certain settings, spread to others. The usual result is trouble for everyone.

During the past seven or eight years, another example of misidentified hysterical behavior has surfaced and again has been bolstered by an invented view of its cause that fits a cultural fashion. This condition is "multiple personality disorder" (MPD, as it has come to be abbreviated). The majority of the patients who eventually receive this diagnosis come to therapists with standard psychiatric complaints, such as depression or difficulty in relationships. Some therapists see much more in these symptoms and suggest to the patient and to others that they represent the subtle actions of several alternative personalities, or "alters," coexisting in the patient's mental life. These suggestions encourage many patients to see their problems in a fresh and, to them, remarkably interesting way. Suddenly they are transformed into odd people with repeated shifts of demeanor and deportment that they display on command.

Sexual politics in the 1980s and 1990s, particularly those connected with sexual oppression and victimization, galvanize these inventions. Forgotten sexual mistreatment in childhood is the most frequently proffered explanation of MPD. Just as an epidemic of bewitchment served to prove the arrival of Satan in Salem, so in our day an epidemic of MPD is used to confirm that a vast number of adults were sexually abused by guardians during their childhood.

Now I don't for a moment deny that children are sometimes victims of sexual abuse or that a behavioral problem originating from such abuse can be a hidden feature in any life. Such realities are not at issue. What I am concerned with here is what has been imagined from these realities and inventively applied to others.

Adults with MPD, so the theory goes, were assaulted as young children by a trusted and beloved person—usually a father, but grandfathers, uncles, brothers, or others, often abetted by women in their power, are also possibilities. This sexual assault, the theory holds, is blocked from memory (repressed and dissociated) because it was so shocking. This dissociating blockade itself—again according to the theory—destroys the integration of mind and evokes multiple personalities as separate, disconnected, sequestered, "alternative" collections of thought, memory, and feeling. These resultant distinct "personalities" produce a variety of what might seem standard psychiatric symptoms—depression, weight problems, panic states, demoralization, and so forth—that only careful review will reveal to be expressions of MPD that is the outcome of sexual abuse.

These patients have not come to treatment reporting a sexual assault in childhood. Only after therapy has promoted MPD behavior is the possibility that they were sexually abused as children suggested to them. From recollections of the mists of childhood, a vague sense of vulnerability may slowly emerge, facilitated and encouraged by the treating group. This sense of vulnerability is thought a harbinger of clearer memories of victimization that, although buried, have been active for decades producing the different "personalities." The long supposedly forgotten abuse is finally "remembered" after months of "uncovering" therapy, during which long conversations by the therapist with "alter" personalities take place. Any other actual proof of the assault is thought unnecessary. Spectral evidence—developed through suggestions and just as irrefutable as that at Salem—once again is sanctioned.

Like bewitchment from Satan's local agents, the idea of MPD and its cause has caught on among large numbers of psychiatrists and psychotherapists. Its partisans see the patients as victims, cosset them in groups, encourage more expressions of "alters" (up to as many as eighty or ninety), and are ferocious toward any defenders of those who they believe are perpetrators of the abuse. Just as the divines of Massachusetts were convinced that they were fighting Satan by recognizing bewitchment, so the contemporary divines—these are therapists—are confident that they are fighting perpetrators of a common expression of sexual oppression, child abuse, by recognizing MPD.

The incidence of MPD has of late indeed taken on epidemic proportions, particularly in certain treatment centers. Whereas its diagnosis was reported fewer than two hundred times from a variety of supposed causes in the past century, it has been applied to more than twenty thousand people in the past decade and largely attributed to sexual abuse.

I have been involved in direct and indirect ways with five such cases in the past year alone. In every one, the very same story has been played out in a stereotyped scriptlike way. In each a young woman with a rather straightforward set of psychiatric symptoms—depression and demoralization—sought help, and her case was stretched into a diagnosis of MPD. Eventually, in each example, an accusation of prior sexual abuse was leveled by her against her father. The accusation developed after months of therapy, first as vague feelings of a dreamlike kind—childhood reminiscences of danger and darkness eventually crystallizing, sometimes "in a flash," into a recollection of father forcing sex upon the patient as a child. No other evidence of these events was presented but the memory, and plenty of refuting testimony, coming from former nursemaids and the mother, was available but dismissed.

On one occasion, the identity of the molester—forgotten for years and now first vaguely and then more surely remembered under the persuasive power of therapy—changed, but the change was as telling about the nature of evidence as was the emergence of the original charge. A woman called her mother to claim that she had come to realize that when she was young she was severely and repeatedly sexually molested by her uncle, her mother's brother. The mother questioned the daughter carefully about the dates and times of these incidents and then set about determining whether they were in fact possible. She soon discovered that her brother was on military service in Korea at the time of the alleged abuse. With this information, the mother went to her daughter with the hope of showing her that her therapist was misleading her in destructive ways. When she heard this new information, the daughter seemed momentarily taken aback but then said, "I see, Mother. Yes. Well, let me think. If your dates are right, I suppose it must have been Dad." And with that, she began to claim that she had been a victim of her father's abusive attentions, and nothing could dissuade her.

The accused men whom I studied, denying the charges and amazed at their source, submitted to detailed reviews of their sexual lives and polygraphic testing to try to prove their innocence and thereby erase doubts about themselves. Professional requests by me to the daughters' therapists for better evidence of the abuse were dismissed as derived from the pleadings of the guilty and scorned as beneath contempt, given that the diagnosis of MPD and the testimony of the patients patently confirmed the assumptions.

In Salem, the conviction depended on how judges thought witches behaved. In our day, the conviction depends on how some therapists think a child's memory of trauma works. In fact, severe traumas are not blocked out by children but remembered all too well. They are amplified in consciousness, remaining like grief to be reborn and reemphasized on anniversaries and in settings that can simulate the environments where they occurred. Good evidence for this is found in the memories of children from concentration camps. More recently, the children of Chowchilla, California, who were kidnapped in their school bus and buried in sand for many hours remembered every detail of their traumatic experience and need psychiatric assistance, not to bring out forgotten material that was repressed but to help them move away from a constant ruminative preoccupation with the experience.

Upon first hearing of these diagnostic formulations (MPD being the result of repressed memories of sexual abuse in childhood), many psychiatrists have fallen back upon what they think is an evenhanded way of approaching it. "The mind is very mysterious in its ways," they say. "Anything is possible in a family." In fact, this credulous stance toward evidence and the failure to consider the alternative of hysterical behaviors and memories are what continue to support this crude psychiatric analysis.

The helpful clinical approach to the patient with putative MPD, as with any instance of hysterical display, is to direct attention away from the behavior—one simply never talks to an "alter." Within a few days of a consistent therapeutic emphasis away from the MPD behavior, it fades, and generally useful psychotherapy on the presenting true problems begins. Real sexual traumas can be dealt with, if they are present, as can the ambivalent and confused feelings that many adults have about their parents.

Similarly, the proper approach to end epidemics of MPD and the assumptions of a vast prevalence of sexual abuse in ordinary families is for psychiatrists to be aware of the potential, whenever we are dealing with hysteria, to mistake it for something else. When it is so mistaken, this can lead to monstrous concepts defended by coincidence, the induction of memories, and a display of "spectral" evidence—all to justify a belief that the community is under siege. This belief, of course, is what releases the power of the witches' court and the lynch mob.

As a corrective, psychiatrists need only review with a patient how the MPD behavior was diagnosed and how the putative memories of sexual abuse were suggested. These practices will eventually be discredited, and this epidemic will end in the same way that the witch trials ended in Salem. But time is passing, many families are being hurt, and confidence in the competence and impartiality of psychiatry is eroding.

Major psychiatric misdirections often share this intimidating mixture of a medical mistake lashed to a trendy idea. Any challenge to such a misdirection must confront simultaneously the professional authority of the proponents and the political power of fashionable convictions. Such challenges are not for the fainthearted or inexperienced. Challengers seldom quickly succeed because they are often misrepresented as ignorant or, in the cant word of our day, uncaring. Each of the three misdirections I have dealt with in this essay ran for a full decade, despite vigorous criticism. Eventually the mischief became obvious to nearly everyone, and fashion moved on to attach itself to something else.

In ten years much damage can be done, and much effort over a longer period of time is required to repair it. Thus, with the mentally ill homeless, only a new crusade and social commitment will bring them adequate help again. Age accentuates the sad caricature of the sexually reassigned and saps their bravado. Some, pathetically, ask about re-reassignment. Groups of parents falsely accused of sexual mistreatment by their grown children are gathering together to fight back in ways that will produce dramatic but distressing spectacles. How good it would have been if in the first place all these misguided programs had been avoided or at least their span abbreviated.

Psychiatry, it needs always to be remembered, is a medical discipline—capable of glorious medical triumphs and hideous medical mistakes. We psychiatrists don't know the secret of human nature. We cannot build a New Jerusalem. But we can teach the lessons of our past. We can describe how our explanations for mental disorders are devised and develop—where they are strong and where they are vulnerable to misuse. We can clarify the presumptions about what we know and how we know it. We can strive within the traditional responsibilities of our profession to build a sound relationship with people who consult us—placing them on more equal terms with us and encouraging them to approach us as they would any other medical specialists, by asking questions and expecting answers, based on science, about our assumptions, practices, and plans. With effort and good sense, we can construct a clinical discipline that, while delivering less to fashion, will bring more to patients and their families.

The American Scholar, 1992

Psychotherapy Awry

Psychiatrists are physicians who treat patients for troubled thoughts, moods, or behavior—sometimes with medicine, sometimes with talk, often with both. Psychotherapy is the term for the talk treatments. It is an indispensable psychiatric skill but differs radically in its attributes from more familiar medical or surgical procedures. Psychotherapy works for patients as an experience—an experience, specifically, of talking and listening to an expert—and by finding, from within that experience, ways to solve a problem.

At its best, psychotherapy helps patients by getting them to reflect on themselves. With psychotherapy, patients can come to appreciate how their own thoughts and attitudes contribute to their troubles. They may find, in counsel with someone they have reason to trust, better approaches to deal with the world.

This fairly rudimentary description, although based on empirical evidence, ignores an awkward inclination of psychotherapy that represents a long-standing problem for psychiatry. Psychotherapists—as they try to grasp the inner world of patients—can easily slip into raw romanticism. The romanticist tendency in psychotherapy is to rely upon feelings for evidence, on metaphors for reality, on inspiration and myth for guidance. Such romanticism has been a recurrent temptation for therapists confronted by patients with perplexing problems.

Among psychiatrists, a long, growling dispute—about twenty years in duration—has been fought and is now ending between romanticists and the empiricists, who insist that all the practices of psychiatry be based upon observation and methodical study of patients. This dispute is ostensibly about psychotherapy but actually is about the proper direction psychiatry itself ought to take. At stake is who will command the future of psychiatry and, more important, how patients will come to be treated.

The empiricists are winning because their approach has expanded, in a clear and gratifying way, our knowledge of mental disorders. The romantics, in my view, are losing not because they fail to provide

18

helpful proposals for psychotherapy. This is their strength. They are losing because, as romantics will, they have become infatuated by their own thought. They claim to know things they never try to prove. They are charmed by novelty and ignore, even disdain, drab facts. More recently, in their thinking they have taken a nightmarish turn toward chaos that has caused patients and their families much suffering.

As someone who trains psychiatrists, I am responsible for explaining these complex matters to students, especially those who, as resident physicians, are entrusting the formative years of their professional lives to me. I want them to understand the issues of the dispute so that they can follow an educational path with a future. For this purpose, case studies or vignettes in which an overemphasis on romantic inspiration led to mistreatment are extremely helpful. A compelling and unusually detailed example of such a case came to my attention when, in the summer of 1992, I received a call from the Board of Registration in Medicine of the Commonwealth of Massachusetts to confer over a complaint of the most serious psychiatric malpractice.

The case in question involved a Cambridge psychiatrist and a Harvard Medical School student who consulted her. Its tragic culmination in the suicide of the medical student, a promising young man, and the exposure of some very strange psychotherapeutic practices on the part of a respected psychiatrist prompted investigation.

The records and depositions I reviewed were remarkable in providing a rare uncensored view of psychotherapy (they are all now public documents, so that no clinical confidences are violated by discussing them here). They disclose how the therapist lost her way. She neglected standard psychiatric practices, adopted views about the patient that were not true, and acted toward him in ways that were, not to put too fine a point on it, not good. The incident reveals just how far from sound judgment romanticized leanings can carry a therapist, and it teaches important lessons about contemporary psychiatry and psychotherapy.

In July 1986 Paul Lozano, an M.D.-Ph.D. student at Harvard Medical School and member of a Mexican American family from El Paso, Texas, sought treatment for depression from Dr. Margaret Bean-Bayog, a school-affiliated psychiatrist. She restricted her evaluation of his condition to the information he could provide. She never attempted to contact any member of his large family for other facts about his background. Indeed, she resisted efforts on their part to reach her. Nonetheless, Dr. Bean-Bayog concluded that his depression—which manifested itself in delusional, self-blaming, and suicidal ideas—was owing to years of sexual abuse by his mother when he was a child. Paul Lozano had no memory of such abuse, but the doctor proposed that strong repression, in response to the shocking experiences, had pushed it beyond his memory's reach.

Dr. Bean-Bayog delegated responsibility for pharmacologic treatment of Paul Lozano's depressive symptoms to another physician, while she herself took up an emotionally evocative psychotherapy with Lozano. She made many efforts to bring to light in him memories of his putative childhood abuse and attempted to induce in him feelings of devotion for her similar to those a two- or three-year-old child might have for his mother.

The patient's state of mind fluctuated during his four years of almost daily psychotherapy with Dr. Bean-Bayog. Depression and suicidal thoughts came and went. He grew dependent on the therapist and frequently expressed his love and need for her.

For a period of time in the midst of this therapy the doctor was overcome by erotic feelings for the patient. She sustained and embellished her feelings by writing elaborate fantasies of sexual play and sadomasochistic encounters with him that had a distinctly pornographic character.

During the course of treatment, Paul Lozano required several admissions to psychiatric hospitals, where the medical staff, particularly at Harvard's McLean Hospital, viewed Dr. Bean-Bayog as overly involved with him. A psychiatrist at McLean warned her on June 23, 1987: "There is an ongoing question about how much his present therapy is supporting him or stirring up almost inconsolable yearnings and conflictual feelings." Dr. Bean-Bayog, however, continued —with some support from her own chosen consultants—to emphasize the themes of maternal sex abuse, the need to bring to light the repressed memories, and the importance of regression to childhood in her treatment.

After four years of this intense therapy, Dr. Bean-Bayog began to separate herself from Paul Lozano and finally did so in the spring of 1990. A stormy four months followed for the patient, whose suicidal thoughts increased and depression worsened. He was seen in several different Massachusetts hospitals; he was eventually treated vigorously for his depression with a combination of antidepressants, lithium, and electroconvulsive therapy. He responded well to this treatment and had two or three months of freedom from his major symptoms. During this time he told his new doctors that he had not been abused by his mother but allowed that he affirmed Dr. Bean-Bayog's assessment because he had been anxious to retain her interest in him.

Lozano turned over to his new doctors letters, photographs, audiotapes, and more than thirty pages of Dr. Bean-Bayog's handwritten sexual fantasies—which he claimed she gave to him—to corroborate what he said was a sexually intimate relationship between them. His new physicians felt obligated to report the possibility of sexual exploitation of the patient to the Massachusetts Board of Registration in Medicine, the body responsible for reviews of physician practice and conduct.

Lozano continued to yearn for Dr. Bean-Bayog. He had misgivings about revealing their intimacies. On April 2, 1991, before the board could finish its investigation, Paul Lozano, injecting himself dozens of times with cocaine, took his own life.

The startling and provocative nature of the evidence, and the nasty suspicions about psychotherapy that it aroused, attracted the attention of the press. Much comment was critical of Dr. Bean-Bayog. But in both Boston and the national press, statements of support for her treatment of Paul Lozano by eminent psychiatrists appeared. Some said that Lozano represented an extremely difficult case and that Dr. Bean-Bayog was justified in using unconventional methods to "keep him alive." Others complained that both the publicity and the board's investigations were conducted in bad faith and that they were sustained because the physician was a woman accused of misdemeanors more often committed by male therapists. Some even proposed that the patient, jealous and angry, was trying to injure Dr. Bean-Bayog—if at first in life, now from the grave.

The magistrate for the board planned a public hearing at which all available documentary evidence of the treatment and the behavior of the physician was to be reviewed. As the psychiatric consultant to the board, I was expected to provide an opinion about the standards of care reflected in Dr. Bean-Bayog's treatment of Paul Lozano. My testimony was to be rebutted by three distinguished Boston psychiatrists. But, on the day before this hearing, Dr. Bean-Bayog relinquished her medical license—for life, as required by law if resignation comes during an investigation. This rendered moot any assessment of her appropriateness as a physician and psychiatrist. The hearing was canceled.

When she resigned, however, Dr. Bean-Bayog gave the local newspapers a distress-filled statement in which she claimed to have been mistreated by the process of investigation and its publicity. She denied any wrongdoing or mismanagement in the Lozano case. She accused the dead patient and his family of "false allegations," the state officials of "overreaction," and the media of "pandering to the public appetite for preposterous, salacious scandal." And there the case rests, except for the later agreement by Dr. Bean-Bayog's insurance company to settle with the Lozano family—who received her malpractice policy's maximum payment of one million dollars.

A talented young student-scientist at the Harvard Medical School is dead. His family, particularly his mother, remains to this day besmirched by the accusations. A physician with a national reputation is disgraced, her medical career snuffed out. Much finger-pointing remains, but newspaper reports state—as in the *Boston Globe* of December 17, 1992—"the issues remain unresolved."

In fact, the issues in this tragic case *are* resolvable—and with ultimate advantage to an understanding of psychiatry. The case itself is quite simply an example of how *not* to practice psychiatry and psychotherapy today. It also shows how certain beliefs and ways of thinking—mostly romanticized in nature—can blind one to reality. The record of Dr. Bean-Bayog's treatment of Paul Lozano is an anthology of professional errors, both of omission and of commission, involving matters of fact, logic, and principle.

The patient suffered from a major depressive illness that was recurrent, severe, and intermittently disruptive of his mood, his capacity to reason, and his behavior. The evidence confirming this opinion is broad and extends from records of the patient's symptoms, the repeated diagnostic assessments by several clinicians, concurring evidence of hospital laboratory tests, some indications that both his mother and brother may also suffer from this illness, and finally Paul

Lozano's positive response to adequate antidepressant medication and electroconvulsive therapy.

Depression of this sort has the ineluctable character of a disease, and eventually it did lead Paul Lozano to suicide. During its reign he suffered the typical mental characteristics of depression, ones that should have directed his treatment—both pharmacologically and psychotherapeutically.

The pharmacologic treatment of major depression has been one of the great achievements of contemporary psychiatry. To be effective, however, it must be sustained and closely linked to the patient's symptoms. Dr. Bean-Bayog relegated this crucial aspect of Paul Lozano's treatment to someone whom she did not inform about her psychotherapeutic program and whom she seldom consulted. Patients with depression respond best to the combination of pharmacotherapy and psychotherapy, but these need to be carefully coordinated, particularly with a seriously ill person.

Paul Lozano would have been a difficult candidate for psychotherapy—especially the emotionally evocative approach Dr. Bean-Bayog decided to employ—because his depression produced profound and persisting despondency, a deprecatory view of himself, muddled thought, and often brittle emotional responses. He was intermittently swept away by delusional beliefs—"I'm a misfit," "I'm a failure," "I'm despised"—and repeatedly became so disorganized in his thinking as to require hospitalization.

Because Paul Lozano suffered from this kind of depression and these symptoms, even a rehabilitative psychotherapy emphasizing support, concentrating on reality, and coordinated with the proper pharmacotherapy would have been a demanding professional challenge. To embed this sort of psychotherapy into his overall treatment, Dr. Bean-Bayog would have had to persuade Paul Lozano of the nature and fluctuating course of his depressive condition and insist that he overcome any reluctance to continue his medications. She would have had to harp on the irrational nature of his beliefs and sustain him in realistic appraisals of himself. She would have had to enlist the assistance of his family and his medical school deans— again surmounting any resistance he might have had to this plan— who needed to understand his changing states of mind so as to support and protect him during the recurrences of his symptoms. She also would have had to appreciate how this illness could render him vulnerable to suggestion and to views of himself of a debasing and self-blaming kind.

Dr. Bean-Bayog did little of this. Instead she steered Paul Lozano into a form of evocative insight psychotherapy—a psychotherapeutic approach derived from psychoanalysis, its prototype. This approach is designed to mobilize strong feelings in the patient under the assumption that it will bring repressed, emotionally charged conflicts to the patient's awareness for resolution.

But Lozano already was disrupted by the intense emotions of his mental illness, which left him as impaired for a review of his past life as he was for appropriately understanding his present life. In *Persuasion and Healing* (1991), their classic and recently republished book on psychotherapy, Drs. Jerome Frank and Julia Frank describe how useful the evocative psychotherapies can be for patients who have some capacity for emotional control and comprehension of reality. Paul Lozano, however, lacked these qualities because of his mental illness. Dr. Bean-Bayog's decision to employ this evocative approach, which she made early on after her initial meetings with him, is at least debatable and should have been monitored for its suitability at regular intervals and abandoned when adverse effects, such as those noted at McLean Hospital, became obvious.

Even if one accepts, for the sake of discussion, Dr. Bean-Bayog's choice of therapy, its features became grotesque. She gave Paul Lozano teddy bears to help his regression to a childlike status, calling them "transitional objects" to aid a bridging in therapy of childhood into adolescence. She wrote him letters and notes bearing messages of love and devotion, such as "I am your Mom," "I love you very much," "I'll never leave you." During the course of this idiosyncratic form of therapy, Dr. Bean-Bayog lost control of both the emotions she evoked in the patient and those she evoked in herself. He began to ask her for sex. She began to write wild sexual fantasies about him.

From the record it is difficult to say who was the initiator of this inappropriate sexual behavior, but clearly the professional boundaries between doctor and patient that were Dr. Bean-Bayog's responsibility to maintain were breached. An uncontrolled, complex personal relationship was launched under the guise of therapy. It not only had damaging effects on Paul Lozano but would have harmed any patient.

Paul Lozano and Dr. Bean-Bayog differed on whether a fully

consummated sexual relationship developed between them. There is no question, however, that Dr. Bean-Bayog engaged in actions that are forms of "courting" behavior. By "courting" psychiatrists mean actions that ordinarily encourage progressively more intimate relations. Dr. Bean-Bayog fostered an erotic atmosphere in her therapy. She permitted Lozano to take playful and provocative photographs of her. She used loving language to describe their relationship in many of the letters she wrote to him. She did not suppress but elaborated her own erotic feelings for him in richly detailed sexual fantasy writing, and she either gave these products to him, as expressions of her longings for him, or did not ensure that the scripts were inaccessible.

Dr. Bean-Bayog later claimed that this writing was her private way of examining her sexual feelings and bringing them under control. Sexual fantasy writing seems more likely to elaborate than to control such feelings. Certainly, it has never been an outlet recommended for therapists who find themselves in Dr. Bean-Bayog's predicament. Imagine how contrary to common sense it would be if the patient angered her and she responded by writing pages of murderous fantasies that she then kept around the office for reference.

Dr. Bean-Bayog made strenuous efforts—in the legal depositions that were to precede the hearing and again during her exchanges with the press—to deny that her sexual feelings, fantasies, and eroticized interactions with the patient were literally "hers." She always insisted that they be called "feelings in the transference/countertransference sense," intending somehow to sanitize her attitudes and behavior with this professional appellation. Yet a feeling generated during therapeutic encounters, and thus legitimately called an aspect of countertransference, is not any less a personal, real, and compelling feeling. Like any other feeling, it is capable of provoking inappropriate behavior and hence from its inception falls to the responsibility of the expert to control. A countertransference source no more justifies acts against the patient's interest than feelings of love or hate generated in other ways.

This justification by theory put up by Dr. Bean-Bayog and her supporters bears a strong resemblance to the argument in the first chapter of *Pickwick Papers*, where Mr. Blotton calls Mr. Pickwick a humbug. He then mollifies the angry crowd of Pickwick's friends by explaining that he did not mean it in the "common sense" but had used the word in its "Pickwickian sense." "Personally," Blotton wanted all to know, "he entertained the highest regard and esteem for the honorable gentleman, he had merely considered him a humbug in a Pickwickian point of view." Dr. Bean-Bayog and her supporters are bona fide members of The Club when they give this Pickwickian construction to countertransference.

The theme of child abuse, particularly the alleged sexual abuse by Paul Lozano's mother, was central to Dr. Bean-Bayog's diagnosis and therapeutic plan. This, it turns out, does not survive close scrutiny. The allegations emerged in a suspicious way and took on quite incredible features. The notion that Paul Lozano was abused by his mother was from the outset a creation by Dr. Bean-Bayog. She came to this diagnosis because she believed that many of his symptoms were those seen in abused people. She never attempted to verify her suspicions with his brothers, sisters, or family physicians. Paul Lozano did not spontaneously report these alleged incestuous encounters. Only after many therapeutic sessions did Dr. Bean-Bayog persuade him to accept this idea. She had to instruct him on the possibility by having him read articles and books—such as *The Courage to Heal* (1988) by Ellen Bass and Laura Davis—that claim (quite without foundation) to know that multiple experiences of heinous and repetitive abuse in childhood and adolescence can be repressed and thus be unavailable to memory.

This concept of repression in child abuse holds that it is possible to live for years with no memory of multiple experiences of violent and defiling abuse at the hands of one's most trusted guardians. Behind this concept is a dramatic, nightmarish, and fundamentally romanticist misdirection of psychotherapeutic thought, for repression on this scale calls for an astonishing power of mind. The concept emerged from anecdotes in the popular—indeed, paperback—press of the 1970s and 1980s. It is implausible on its face, lacks confirmation by research, and, as Dr. Bean-Bayog did, is usually proposed to patients during therapy without any effort to check any facts. A belief in all-powerful repression often contributes, much as it did here, to redirecting treatment away from real problems as well as to isolating the patient from the natural supports of his family.

Eventually Paul Lozano did begin to report recollections of sexual encounters with his mother, but they took on progressively exotic form, including memories of sex during diaper changes at age two. Detailed remembrances from so early in life are, to put it gently, dubious in the extreme. The fact that Lozano eventually claimed to have them strongly suggests that he did not repress a series of shocking sexual encounters with his mother. It suggests instead that his "memories" were either induced in him (a self-blaming emotionally dependent patient) by suggestions from his trusted therapist or were, as he later claimed, reported by him as a means of retaining Dr. Bean-Bayog's interest and affection. In any case, the evidence in this record for sexual abuse of Paul Lozano by his mother is far weaker than the evidence that Dr. Bean-Bayog was sexually involved with him.

The reasons why Dr. Bean-Bayog's treatment of her patient went radically wrong go beyond these particulars. Throughout the treatment of Paul Lozano the major deficiency was an extended absence of good judgment on the part of Dr. Bean-Bayog. This was displayed in many ways. Chief among them were Dr. Bean-Bayog's overconfidence in her first impressions, her credulity toward theory, her stubbornness in the face of criticism, her rashness with intimacy, and, in the end, her willingness to give up her life's work—a form of professional suicide—rather than explain her practice to the public.

What perverted this physician's judgment? The answer to that question emerges from a study of the language and statements of belief that fill both the case notes and many of the legal depositions of Dr. Bean-Bayog and her consultants.

Most of this is cast, right from the start, in the interpretive idiom of psychodynamic metaphors. Disconcertingly absent is simple description, ordinary exposition of the personal experience of this young student and his family, of the unembellished, mundane humanness of their lives and of their places in this world. Everything is given a dubious "depth" of sexual coloration; all is couched in psychological officialese: transference and countertransference, repression, transitional objects, symbol, and metaphor.

Even Paul Lozano's suicide attempts were explained to the patient by a sexual metaphor. One of the consultants who was asked by Dr. Bean-Bayog to see Paul Lozano during a hospital stay wrote, after his visit with the patient: "Through our conversation he and I were able to relate this [suicidal behavior] to masturbatory excitement in which one retains and maintains control of one's own pleasure, thrill and sexual excitement: control over life and death . . . and freedom in the sense of having his own life in his hands."

Nothing in the Lozano case was seen for what it was, to be judged for itself. Paul Lozano's self-blame was not a symptom of a depressive illness but rather a sign of repressed sex abuse. Dr. Bean-Bayog's pornographic writings were not a surrender to impulse and a breakdown in professional distance but an expression of the countertransference. Everything, even death, was something else.

Officialese has done here what officialese always does—replaced observation, corrupted judgment, and, on more than one occasion, deprived its agent, Dr. Bean-Bayog, of the capacity to see the obvious. The blinding qualities of ambiguous language, murky thought, and unexamined belief were fundamental to all the trouble that followed. Romanticism had run riot, justifying every excess.

All patients requiring psychotherapy have a similar debilitating and distressing sense of confusion and incompetence. Jerome Frank has aptly called their state of mind demoralization—a combination of discouragement and perceived loss of self-efficiency. People with such symptoms will be uneasy about approaching a psychotherapist for help if they think an experience in any way resembling Paul Lozano's is what they risk.

There were no obvious warnings to Paul Lozano or his family that he was in danger of mistreatment. He was not, of course, consulting a fringe therapist but a reputable psychiatrist, one associated with the Harvard Medical School. What Dr. Bean-Bayog did seemed to be supported by other psychiatric consultants. When Paul Lozano became acutely ill, he was taken to well-known hospitals and cared for by experienced staffs—on one occasion, he was visited by the chief of the service.

After the tragic outcome of the Lozano case, there were psychiatrists who were willing to state for the local and national press that nothing was wrong with Dr. Bean-Bayog's treatment. The case, they claimed, was just a very tough one. If only people were sophisticated in psychological matters and looked at the elements "in context," they would see that the difficulties lay not with the course of treatment but with the patient and (more subtly implied) with the family. "Providing psychotherapeutic treatment is not like making tollhouse cookies," the then president of the Massachusetts Psychiatric Society told the Boston press.

Such statements represented a hasty and reflexive defense of Dr.

Bean-Bayog—the group protecting a challenged member—rather than a thoughtful critique of a psychiatric practice to help people understand what happened to Paul Lozano. This was indeed a tough case, as the record shows. But then many psychiatric cases are tough. That is why specialists with advanced training are needed. Better explanations, not professional sarcasm, are required to resolve the concerns this case raises and to reassure people considering psychotherapy.

Not only is psychotherapy not the making of Toll House cookies; it is, most distinctly, not a creative art form. It isn't a mystery play; it isn't a secret initiation. It is neither a romance nor a rite. It is instead a professional action that fits into other aspects of patient care according to empirical psychiatric principles that can be made clear to anyone.

In fact, there should be no mystery about what psychiatrists can do. They can heal the symptoms of some diseases; guide and protect a patient from the promptings of temperament; interrupt destructive behaviors such as addiction; and help patients rethink their assumptions so as to enhance their capacity to deal with the present and the future.

Psychotherapy plays a role in every one of these actions by explaining the nature of mental symptoms, resolving misunderstandings, or encouraging more constructive life strategies. It helps to restore the patient's sense of self-efficiency. Usually the patient presents the psychiatrist with a combination of problems, as did Paul Lozano, and needs a coordinated treatment plan in which psychotherapy is embedded.

To return to the comments from Boston, it is revealing to view the elements of treatment in context. Psychotherapy does not, after all, occur in an intellectual vacuum. The particular context of any example of psychotherapy can be gleaned from its main preoccupations. A relentless interest in sex and an unbalanced emphasis on deficiencies of the patient's family rather than on any of the family's strengths usually indicate a tight coupling of the psychotherapy to Freudian psychoanalytic thought.

Although Freud's fame is secure on other grounds, his followers, it is now becoming plain, often overvalued his nineteenth-century Teutonic vision of an irresistible force upon humanity—here tied to the sexual libido that Freud made central to mental life and personal development. In many ways Freud belongs to the family of monorail thinkers that can claim Karl Marx. Freud added a dynamic unconscious running on libidinous energy to all those other impersonal and ineluctable forces—history, economics, the nation-state, and so on—identified east of the Rhine as governing our fate and to which we are but putty.

Such a key to human nature, of course, appealed to psychotherapists (and to a multitude of other articulate people in the twentieth century who joined the psychoanalytic movement and transformed it from a clinical proposal into a highly romanticized social doctrine). It provided—as Karl Popper condemned in Hegel—"a quick initiation into the deeper secrets of this world [without] the laborious technicalities of science which after all may only disappoint by lack of power to unveil all mysteries."

But this intellectual romanticism just won't fit with the empirical knowledge that is advancing the practice of psychiatry today. Single-minded, overconfident, and derived from an outmoded philosophical tradition, it has been the context for many examples of misguided and interminable therapy such as that given Paul Lozano.

Efforts to force psychotherapy along paths suggested by some all-encompassing vision of human nature are being replaced by an approach that develops psychotherapeutic aims from verifiable observations of the patient and the actual circumstances of his or her life. Since mental disorders come in several forms, they derive from the endless sources of trouble presented by life—including but not limited to those identified by Freud. For any particular patient, though, all sources of trouble—losses, burdens, illness, temperament, habitual attitudes, or simply fears that the future may replay the past—must be explored and *verified* by the therapist, preferably before therapy is launched but definitely as it proceeds and new facts come to light.

Such explorations, in which the patient actively participates, can certainly be laborious and time-consuming—as my resident physicians remind me—and are unlikely to unveil the secrets of human nature. But they will reveal the actual problems patients face and the way to combine the several treatments they need. For their and psychiatry's purposes, that is plenty.

Some rather simple principles of procedure are now, reassuringly, standard in psychotherapy. Early in the course of treatment the psychiatrist should lay out for the patient the logical therapeutic and prognostic implications that emerge from a diagnosis. The beliefs underlying a psychotherapeutic plan should be brought to light and scrutinized by the therapist and the patient together in order to decide just how good these are as working assumptions in the patient's case. As the doctor delineates the treatment plan, he or she should describe the patient's role and responsibilities in it. Such "role induction"— to use the professional term—clarifies the mutual expectations for patient and therapist. It makes clear what behavior is intolerable in its course. Finally, if recovery is unexpectedly slow, either the patient or the therapist should request a second opinion. Then the records can be reviewed, the implications of lack of progress explored, and the course of treatment realigned.

There is something more here, though, than principles for effective practice. These briefly sketched points represent the operational implications for the shift—indeed, the sea change—from romanticism to empiricism in psychiatry. The inscrutable all-knowing man behind the couch is disappearing from therapy just as sexual metaphor and Greek myth are disappearing from psychiatric explanations.

In their place is an appreciation that mental life is as open to empirical assessment as are other aspects of the world. Empiricism prompts psychiatrists and patients alike to work with what can be observed and confirmed—emphasizing what we know and how we know it. It indicates how decisions for treatment are made, how their strengths are reviewed, and how their errors are corrected. It does not exclude inspiration but keeps it within bounds.

Empiricism is changing the way psychiatrists think and talk. This is a slow process, and vestigial elements of romantic excess still intrude—as, for example, when every cruel person is called sadistic and every prideful person a narcissist. But the fears that this shift of emphasis toward empiricism would lead to an abandonment of concern for human feelings and their dynamic interactions have proved groundless. Psychiatrists with an empirical approach are vitally interested in the patient's thoughts and feelings. They know that these mental experiences reveal the burdens and impairments of a patient in need of treatment. In fact, by forsaking the false light of metaphor and myth, psychiatrists have gained a clearer sense of the attributes of patients.

The concern that only biological information and not psychological information would interest the empiricists in psychiatry has been dispelled. The shift from a romantic to an empirical emphasis is not a move from dynamic psychiatry to biological psychiatry. Rather, empirical information adds facts to a dynamic understanding. Empirical psychology has provided information about temperament and drive that illuminates the distinctions among people in their emotional response to particular ordeals and guides the choice of treatment for alcohol and drug addiction.

The move away from romanticism and toward empiricism is a shift that brings psychiatry closer to contemporary medicine and to the beneficial ways of thought advancing medicine today. We psychiatrists may lose the authority that any cloak of mystery brought us and certainly shall find ourselves more exposed to sharp questioning from patients, their families, and a critical public. If, however, we respond as physicians committed to explaining our work and eliminating errors from it, the prospects for patients will improve. Psychotherapy, properly construed and properly conducted, will be better understood by everyone and will come to have a settled place among the treatments of human illness. *The American Scholar, 1994*

What's the Story?

I teach psychiatry to medical students and residents by emphasizing fundamental matters such as defining terms, describing symptoms, and reviewing concepts—the ABCs, you might say, of this medical specialty. I choose this approach because, as all teachers know, most mistakes are with fundamentals. And, perhaps more important, what makes a point fundamental makes it interesting.

Although I have taught this subject this way for more than twenty-five years, every spring I fret about the introductory lecture on psychiatry to the Johns Hopkins University medical students. I don't worry about my grasp of the material; I have covered it before. I don't worry about capturing the students' interest because anybody can be lively when talking about insanity. My fear is that I will mishandle an almost inevitable argument with some members of the class over how to think about mental illness and that this will sour the rest of our time together. As it turns out, the issues I address are not simple. They challenge a deeply rooted supposition about psychiatric patients which students have absorbed from the popular culture and which they are loath to surrender.

This supposition holds that psychiatric patients are fundamentally alike because people are similar in sentiments and psychological vulnerabilities. Their mental disorders therefore vary only in degree, not in kind. Any distinctions in the symptoms of mental disorders depend upon burdens imposed by the biographical events, life patterns, and social settings in which people do differ. This kindly intended "fellowship of mankind" idea that many of my students hold is one of those half-truths that cause me more trouble than any flat-out error.

The facts are that, although some patients derive their mental distress from life situations, many patients suffer from symptoms that are entirely distinct from normal psychological states, symptoms that rest upon bodily disease. Teaching students how to make this distinction and to appreciate its importance in treatment, prognosis, and research is the mission of my department.

I always show students a patient with this first lecture. At this point

I am not trying to explain much. I just want to present an afflicted person and let his or her disarray speak for itself. This modest aim seldom runs smoothly.

On a typical occasion, I was sitting before one hundred students with a woman whom I encouraged to describe her thoughts and feelings. She stated that she was frightened because one of the NASA satellites had been preempted by the Freemasons to record her every movement. She believed that the satellite had been equipped to beam down an invisible but powerful ray, forcing upon her blasphemous thoughts. She rejected any suggestion from me that this might be her imagination or the remnant of some nightmare. She was in the hospital because she called the FBI repeatedly. She wanted to meet the president and have him put a stop to this business.

With such a set of symptoms I felt safe in saying that she had an incapacitating mental disorder such as schizophrenia. After thanking her and helping her return to the ward, I began discussing her state. I noted that she was not afflicted by NASA or the Masons but by a delusion—an idiosyncratic, incorrigible, preoccupying false belief. I parsed that definition, emphasizing that psychiatrists underline the idiosyncratic features of delusional false beliefs to differentiate delusions from mistaken assumptions that might derive from a patient's social group or education. I emphasized that this helped distinguish the symptoms of an illness from ordinary errors.

A student shot up his hand. With disdain, he said, "That poor woman's beliefs would only be called false if you took a narrow view of them. You should consider them within her life of poverty, chaos, and neglect. Then you would see them differently. She developed thoughts about NASA and the Masons to make sense out of a frightening and perplexing world."

The student, a college anthropology major, elaborated on this theme, saying that the false beliefs of this person served the same function as the cultural myths and beliefs of other civilizations that give life sense and purpose in the face of mysterious natural forces. "Those beliefs," he said, "certainly are adaptive, and no one thinks of them as symptoms of derangement or entitles them 'false.'"

I have learned not to interrupt when a student runs an indictment of me as both insensitive and narrow minded. To do so would only encourage a glimmering notion among the other students that perhaps I *am* a social oppressor, placing an additional burden on the patient by calling her mentally ill.

But as I listened to his version—with its fashionable multicultural stance toward both the patient and me—I knew that I would have to put aside anything else I planned to discuss that day and concentrate on the issue of story explanations in psychiatry. The student was attempting to tell a story about this patient that, to him, made sense of her symptoms. If I hoped to teach him or anyone else in the class what they needed to learn, we first had to consider how stories worked sometimes to help and sometimes to hinder psychiatry and whether a story provided an adequate understanding of this patient.

So what's the story? Psychiatrists often use a story to make a patient's symptoms intelligible—capturing the array of symptoms within a narrative of settings and sequential events in the patient's life. The story is thus one of the clinical "tools" of psychiatrists. In fact, all psychotherapists eventually compose with the patient's cooperation some kind of story—a chronicle that reveals how psychological symptoms arise when such motivations as hopes, commitments, preferences, and fears collide with reality.

The "motive" theme distinguishes the psychiatric story from the standard medical case report, in which the onset and progress of symptoms are also described. The medical report is an account of nature's power over human life through infections, neoplasms, genes, and the like. In case after case, medical reports describe the stereotypical progressions and characteristic effects of these natural processes.

The typical psychiatric story, however, replaces nature's power with human motives and suggests that distressing mental states emerge when a patient faces some conflict between purposes and events in his or her life, between expectations and reality. The story provides, through its narrative power, all listeners, especially the patient, with a compelling sense of insight into the symptoms as they relate to this conflict.

Psychiatric stories also work to persuade people to alter their habitual thoughts and behaviors—another distinguishing characteristic. Nowhere is this method more vigorously employed than in the therapeutic efforts of members of Alcoholics Anonymous. The central theme of the AA story is the bondage to alcohol—a powerful metaphor that weaves the different stories of drunken revelry into a common image, encouraging any new member of the group to begin to move from addiction to sobriety as one might move from slavery to freedom.

The narrative power of a story, however, can, as I have learned from so many encounters with students, blind everyone to other explanations of the patient's symptoms, such as the effects of disease or the contribution of a patient's temperament. I was a student myself—an undergraduate, in fact—when I was first struck by the power of a story to create a dubious insight.

One bright day in the late 1940s, the poet John Ciardi substituted for our instructor, Mr. Ludwig, in English A, the freshman composition course at Harvard College required of those who had misspent their high school years and needed help learning to express themselves. Ciardi was not prepared to work on elementary matters that we, the backward freshmen, needed. He wished to show us the future as he saw it written out in Sigmund Freud's monograph on Leonardo da Vinci.

Ciardi enjoyed himself that day. He exuberantly explained how Leonardo's dream about a great bird beating its tail against his face when he was a baby was a prototypical Freudian dream. As Freud explained them, dreams hid from consciousness by representing, in a disguise, an unacceptable impulse—in this instance, Leonardo's homosexual urges. "That long tail, don't you know."

Ciardi believed that the Freudian "discoveries" of dream mechanisms and the dynamic unconscious unveiled the hidden motivations that lay at the heart of all human actions (not just pathological ones) and so by extension could explain the motives behind any of our behaviors. He accepted Freud's view that the key to Leonardo's difficulties in finishing some of his monumental projects was hidden behind this childhood fantasy. Ciardi became irritated when a couple of us—with little more than an offhand reluctance to accept his point without more evidence—challenged the argument. We thought the issue at hand had to do with the use of symbol and metaphor as explanations.

Several days before, Mr. Ludwig had emphasized, when teaching about figures of speech, that metaphorical images used by writers revealed as much about the authors' preoccupations as about the things they portrayed. That was, of course, a typical freshman composition concept, right from the syllabus you might say, but it was an idea that at the moment was big news to me. It was an "Aha!" moment, illuminating important distinctions in the images and language, such as those differentiating classical from romantic poetry.

And that's what we said to Ciardi. Freud has extrapolated a sexual image from a dream. That action, we suggested, may tell more about Freud's mind than about Leonardo's. But Ciardi had not come to listen to such talk. For him, Freud was a wonder and a source, not an author to be examined. "You must have some unresolved sexual problem," he said to me in particular and thus provided my first (and far from last) exposure to the repression-resistance stratagem psychiatric storytellers tend to use against their critics. The class broke up into those persuaded by Ciardi's argument and those unpersuaded, with me a highly irritated member of the latter.

Ciardi was an established poet, an illustrious member of the English Department, a translator of Dante, a practiced expert on symbol and metaphor. Mr. Ludwig, I am sure, thought he was favoring us that day by finding such a distinguished replacement. But why did this gifted man come to have such confidence in Freud that he failed to work with what he knew from his own profession? What prompted him to bully us, the strugglers with language before him, rather than win us round with more information?

The story he accepted overlooked more plausible explanations for Leonardo's difficulties—especially Leonardo's efforts to push the artistic techniques of his time to the limit. Ciardi had found, within the license of metaphor, a warranty for dubious opinions. On many occasions since then with students of my own, I have been reminded of John Ciardi and how he was bedazzled by narrative.

This idea—that stories are compelling and therefore must be employed carefully in psychiatry—lay behind my argument with the beginning student who found in a story a way to make sense of the delusional patient. This student was disagreeing with me over what was important. I claimed that the patient's beliefs were delusional and therefore marks of schizophrenia—a disease that called for special kinds of help and for medication. He thought that her ideas were adaptive responses to a life of adversity, which might disappear if she found some understanding and support from me in facing those adversities.

The student has mighty champions on his side. Freud would be there. He said: "That delusional formation which we take to be the pathological product is in reality an attempt at recovery, a process of reconstruction." Carl Jung is definitely in his corner. He said: "Closer study of [deluded individuals] will show that these patients are consumed by a desire to create a new world system . . . that will enable them to simulate unknown psychic phenomena and so adapt themselves to their own world."

These old warriors and their views are hardly unfamiliar to me. In fact, I know their value in enlarging the scope of psychiatry and in appreciating some of the responses of patients. Prior to their proposals, psychiatrists may have concentrated too much on description, diagnosis, and physical treatment of the patients in their care and may have slipped into habits of disregard for them and for the circumstances of their lives. These masters of psychotherapy encouraged psychiatrists to emphasize that patients are people—not simply objects of nature but vital subjects like the rest of us with aims, purposes, hopes, and fears—in need of aid.

The problem was that these champions tended to overreach themselves. They extended their conceptions about psychiatric disorders so far as to depict them all as expressions no different in kind from the rest of human psychological life. In so doing, it must be said, they played a bit fast and loose with evidence in developing their opinions about human nature and the provocations of mental illness.

Freud was not bashful about this extension. He noted that "psychoanalysis [restricted to] psychiatry would never have drawn the attention of the intellectual world to it or won it a place in the 'history of our times.' This result was brought about by the relation of psychoanalysis to normal, not to pathological, mental life." And on another occasion, he wrote: "If we can temper the severity of the requirements of historical-psychological investigation we may be able to clarify problems which . . . merit our attention." Jung was unambiguous about his intentions and methods when he said: "I can only make direct statements, only 'tell stories'; whether or not the stories are 'true' is not the problem. The only question is whether what I tell is *my* fable, *my* truth."

Freud and Jung were certainly candid about their methods and aims. They were the most vocal proponents of the idea that all psychological symptoms arise from a patient's encounter with life and can be understood like the outcome of a story. They were also certain that such symptoms would dissipate when their provocations were understood and the patients—with the assistance of psychotherapists—found more adaptive ways of responding to their problematic lives.

These assumptions of Freud and Jung represent—as Auden said about Freudianism—"a whole climate of opinion." Jung has emphasized the importance of this aspect of his stories. A conceptual framework—that which he calls *his* truth and which comprises, of course, his assumptions—lies behind the tales he tells and makes them persuasive to him and to his patients. Psychiatric stories announce an author and what that author thinks. My medical student's multicultural story and Ciardi's claims for Leonardo rest on their beliefs, their assumptions about how people behave, *their* truth.

Imagination and reality often coalesce in the assumptions of psychotherapists. The assumptions foster the stories the therapists tell and provide justification for claiming some events to be psychologically important and others trivial in a patient's biography. And because the eventual story is a re-creation of what the psychotherapist assumes, its very composition—the fitting of events together in a narrative form—reinforces the confidence of the therapist in the correctness of the climate of opinion from which he or she began. In psychiatry, this "hermeneutic round"—from assumptions to stories to assumptions confirmed for the more confident composition of further stories—can sweep hesitancy aside and produce a dominating orthodoxy in which all psychiatric disorders are seen as emerging from the inherent potentials of human beings when faced with adverse circumstances or unfriendly associates.

I was first plunged into the steamy climate of this orthodoxy by two teachers at Harvard Medical School. They were professors of psychiatry who worked with narrative in explaining the illnesses of their patients and, in the process, revealed implications embedded in their own assumptions.

Dr. Elvin Semrad was the director of residency training at the Massachusetts Mental Health Center. He was a short, stocky man with a distant manner toward students. He had, however, a way that urged patients suffering from schizophrenia or manic-depression to talk about themselves. He encouraged them to describe their lives and their responses to the crises of the moment. His aim was to suggest to them (and those of us listening in) how they had found, in their disordered mental states, an escape from problems that beset them.

The patients were comforted by Dr. Semrad's attention. They resembled ordinary people in many ways. That was his point: much that is normal is to be found in patients with serious mental illnesses.

But that also was the problem. Dr. Semrad made so much of patients' normality that why they were ill became less obvious. These patients were hearing voices; they were driven by emotional states that did not abate; they had idiosyncratic false beliefs. They were different in some significant way, despite the many normal features they retained. That difference is what made them patients, and that difference needed explanation. Dr. Semrad's skill at unfolding their personal stories, and, while doing so, obviously comforting and encouraging them, permitted everyone to brush by that point.

After Dr. Semrad's death, admiring students gathered his remarks about patients into a book—a collection of maxims, mottoes, and adages. Stories usually produce aphoristic generalizations—words of wisdom—rather than scientific laws and hypotheses. Like the story itself, aphorisms tend to assert rather than prove a viewpoint. These particular maxims, however, are most useful because they demonstrate what Dr. Semrad believed—the assumptions from which he worked—and how these particular beliefs shaped the stories he told and the teaching he gave.

Examples of Dr. Semrad's axioms found in the book include: "Psychotic patients are no different than we are, just a little crazier"; "We're just big messes trying to help bigger messes and the only reason we can do it is that we've been through it before and have survived"; "Don't get set on curing her, but on understanding her. If you understand, and she understands what you understand, then cure will follow naturally." Dr. Semrad assumed—fundamentally from his allegiance to the story method and the prevailing Freudian climate—that the remarkable symptoms of the mentally ill were exaggerations of universal human problems and that these symptoms would disappear when everybody got the story right and set about helping the patient find a better way of adapting to life.

Dr. Semrad influenced a generation of psychiatrists, making them aware of the humanity of their patients, and for this he is warmly remembered. However, not only did he fail to differentiate what was wrong with the patients, he skipped past this question with a set of plausible assumptions and epigrams that implied that every patient, like some lost child, was simply expressing distress in the only way he or she knew how. Dr. Semrad thought that what psychiatrists needed to help patients was not more knowledge of their disorders but more feeling for their plight.

My other teacher, Dr. Ives Hendrick, was a different sort of man. By the time I met him, he had let himself go. He looked seedy in a three-piece suit, down the front of which were food stains and burns from cigarette ashes. As he smoked and talked, he would flick his cigarette without drawing it far from his lips so that a regular flow of ashes spilled onto his chest and abdomen.

Dr. Hendrick's skill was in his grasp of theory. He could apply the orthodox explanation to any symptom, for he was saturated in the Freudian assumptions. He worked backward from the patient's symptoms composing a story and weaving the symptoms into it, a story in which the patient could be pictured as attempting to adapt to stresses found in sexual conflicts and generating a psychological disorder in the process.

I once presented, to a hospital conference Dr. Hendrick was leading, a recently married young woman who was suffering from a classical condition. She was anxious about swallowing her food and felt that a portion often stuck like a lump in her throat. This condition, which goes under the term *globus hystericus,* is often a problem for individuals of an introverted and perfectionist temperament and resembles other hypochondriacal anxieties over bodily function in both its characteristics and its provocations.

Dr. Hendrick saw a symbol in this patient's symptom that fit into his assumptions about the nature of mental disorder. He interrupted my presentation by stating that, as a case of globus hystericus, this patient's problem was obviously conflict over oral sex and that the treatment plan should consist of trying to have her see this problem in the same way he did. He made these comments calmly to the audience of some ten to fifteen social workers and other counselors, all the while puffing on his cigarette and flicking ashes onto his vest.

His opinion was greeted with solemn noddings of heads by everyone in the room. I was floored. Was I really hearing a proposal at Harvard Medical School in Boston that would fit right into the sexual banter of my guttersnipe friends back home in Lawrence? Did the sexual images and obsessions of adolescence reach so far that even Harvard medical professors couldn't resist them?

I was also embarrassed for the patient. The proposal struck such a coarse, degrading note. Here was this grubby guy pontificating to a room full of somber and rather condescending people, all of whom acted as if some great truth had been uttered—before, I should say, an attempt had been made to interview the patient and consider what things other than sex might be troubling her. No duty to fact could withstand their ardor for metaphor.

These two psychiatrists were narrators of mental disorder and actually had similar assumptions about the sources of psychiatric symptoms. They were both members of the Boston Psychoanalytic Institute, which was devoted to promulgating an orthodox Freudian perspective on mental life. True enough, they began at opposite ends of the story. Dr. Semrad began with the person and never quite reached the illness, having been waylaid by the fascinating details of normality. Dr. Hendrick began with the symptom and never quite reached the person, having recast the patient's worries into a symbol of carnal conflict and letting it go at that.

Neither doctor, though, seemed baffled by anything about the patients. Both were confident that the explanations their stories provided were adequate. They were certain about their underlying assumptions and never questioned them. They presumed that the life events they emphasized for the patients were the most important features to understand. Eventually, they produced a psychiatry of categorical mistakes and narrative error, primarily because of the assumptive world to which they were too faithful and in which their final conclusions were hopelessly embedded.

In one sense, the Freudian era is over. The "climate of opinion" that envisaged human beings as puppets of the unconscious manipulated by such stirrings of sexual conflict as Oedipal complexes, castration fears, and penis envy no longer dominates the psychiatric profession. But, in another sense, an essential idea—of which Freudianism is simply one of the examples—lives on in the views and practices of many psychotherapists who restrict their explanations to the story.

These therapists assume that human sentiments are so alike, human vulnerabilities so identical, and human expressions of distress so similar that any psychological disorder must be an adaptive response to a misadventure, trial, or burden. The presumption is: where there is present smoke of mental illness, there must be, at the least, past fire of mishandling and probably mistreatment that distorted the natural course of the patient's psychological development. If these provocations are unappreciated or unremembered by the patient, their implications and existence must be revealed to him or her through psychotherapy. The biography of the patient, therefore, must be explored until the damaging events are discerned and the real story behind the mental disorder—sometimes presented as a drama starring those quasi persons, id, ego, and superego, that Freud invented—is understood by everyone.

Great implications that extend into attitude and action are tied to the view that psychiatric patients are essentially the same. For example, as the medical student rejects the categorical features of schizophrenia in the patient I presented and sees her delusions as a natural effort to adapt to life's adversities, that student must at least suspect the parents and other relatives of the patient as potential sources of the adversities that beset her and, *even before evidence can emerge*, will approach them in a suspicious way. Psychiatric stories based on the assumption that only life's burdens can produce disorder have in the past led to depictions of parents of schizophrenic patients as "double binding" or "schizophrenogenic" and parents of patients with early infantile autism as generating the condition in their offspring through cold and obsessional child-rearing practices.

These false views have been disastrous to everyone. They have put therapists and families at odds with one another at the very time when they need to cooperate in the treatment and rehabilitation of these afflicted patients. As well, the therapists' opinions delayed research into these conditions for years. By mistakenly presuming that the causes of these conditions were known and the family complicit in provoking them, physicians undermined any chance of a cooperative alliance with the family in research.

The assumption that something *must* have happened if a mental disorder is present has provided an entry for zealots and charlatans into psychiatry. There have been Marxist therapists, feminist therapists, and sociobiological therapists—all attempting to write their presumptions into an explanation for mental disorders without a comprehensive study of the conditions themselves. In the past few years, as we all might have expected from the presumption that only life's burdens can produce disorder, patients have been told by therapists that their mental ailments were expressions of (you name it) infantile sexual assaults, satanic cult abuse, space alien abduction, or even irritating remnants of problems "unsolved" in some prior life in other centuries. This is the story explanation gone wild, with immeasurable damage to public confidence in the standards of practice represented by psychiatry and psychotherapy.

It is simply not true that mental disorders are all of one kind, varying in degree but not in nature. To make this clear, psychiatrists must confront the half-truth that the kindly intended "caring" fellowship-of-mankind idea represents. Some mental disorders are expressions of bodily disease. Others represent the effects of body-based drives either innate, such as hunger and sex, or acquired, such as the addictions. Some disorders are, like grief, the understandable outcome of life events. Other conditions depend upon vulnerabilities within the patient's constitution, such as emotional instability or mental retardation. Psychiatrists are responsible for the treatment of all these different conditions and must distinguish them to do so.

There should be no mystery about the treatments these conditions entail. Psychiatrists seek to cure diseases, interrupt behaviors, comfort the grieving, strengthen and guide the vulnerable.

The psychiatric story—a narrative recounting of how a person's hopes, desires, purposes, and constraints influenced the direction of his or her life—fits into every one of these treatments, both those that rest on medicine and those that depend on talk. It provides a natural and coherent context within which to appreciate patients and their troubles. An understanding of context—the way this individual is unique even as he or she suffers from symptoms common to all who have this particular mental illness—illuminates the diagnostic task, transforming it from a simple process of attaching a label to a patient into something more like portraying a person's misfortune.

Narrative details arouse everyone's compassion for the patient and mediate the alliance between patient and physician. Stories uncover how patients' character and life plans were affected by their disorder and what responses come most easily to them as they and their physicians attempt to deal with it. But—and this is the big *but*—the context of a life should not be confused with the cause of all mental disorders or made the sole focus of therapeutic attention as though guidance were always synonymous with cure.

The story method and psychotherapy work together most straight-forwardly when the patient's problems truly are context-driven and tied to universal human themes—grief from loss, fear from threat, demoralization from failure or rejection. Apt stories that provide an empathic understanding of these themes are as many as the predica-ments in life and the individuals who encounter them. Freud and Jung identified some of these predicaments, but most of them are specific to the patient at hand and come to light in the midst of psychotherapy, where the patient and the therapist work together to get the story right.

Story-driven psychotherapy also is a crucial part of the rehabilita-tion of patients afflicted by psychiatric symptoms from other sources, such as disease. For example, patients with manic-depression need medication for their illness, but they also need psychotherapy to understand their affliction and to find ways to live effectively despite its intermittent disruptive symptoms. Any psychiatrist with a knowl-edge of this illness, as well as the story of its specific intrusions into the life of an individual, can and should provide both the medicine and the psychotherapy to the patient simultaneously.

Psychiatrists who try to work without the story forgo a vital way of appreciating their patients' predicaments. However, psychiatrists who rely only on stories to explain mental disorders often misin-terpret and misrepresent them. If these psychiatrists teach others to impose narrative solutions upon clinical problems arbitrarily, pre-maturely, and without attention to evidence, they will cheat their students of the knowledge and experience needed to join the group advancing this medical specialty in the future.

All these thoughts are at work in my argument with the medical stu-dent at the first lecture. I am far from denying that story-based ideas have helped psychiatric practice. What I am saying is that sometimes the story is a fable and—despite the kindest of intentions—does not fit as an explanation. For example, when we are confronted by a patient suffering from the symptoms of schizophrenia, the patient's domination by illness can be obscured for a student who reaches into the contemporary fashions for a story that will make the patient's confusing presentation intelligible. The patient has become a charac-ter in a tale the student can imagine rather than a person afflicted with a condition the student must come to learn.

All medical students, and eventually the public, need to realize that stories are helpful tools in psychiatry. But if used without reflection on their potential to become myths, medically authorized stories can produce a prolonged misdirection for everyone—doctor, patient, and family alike. Physicians, because they can do much harm with the wrong story, are duty-bound—in ways that poets are not—to check the story against the facts.

Although my first lecture often is disrupted, and even occasionally produces more heat than light, there are other lectures to come and clinical experiences on the wards that I go through with students over the course of their education. Eventually, this teaching, tying the explanations and the treatments of mental disorders together and indicating how our narrative instincts can lead us astray, wins out with most of them—not with all, I have to say—because the patients are around to remind us continually of the numerous ways we can get things wrong and, happily, the illuminating occasions when things do go right.   *The American Scholar*, 1995

How Psychiatry Lost Its Way

"The desire to take medicine," noted the great Johns Hopkins physician William Osler a hundred years ago, "is one feature that distinguishes man, the animal, from his fellow creatures." In today's consumer culture, this desire is hardly restricted to people with physical conditions. Psychiatric patients who in the past would bring me their troublesome mental symptoms and their worries over the possible significance of those symptoms now arrive in my office with diagnosis, prognosis, and treatment already in hand.

"I've got adult attention deficit disorder," a young man informs me, "and it's hindering my career. I need a prescription for Ritalin." When I inquire as to the source of his analysis and its proposed solution, he tells me he has read about the disorder in a popular magazine, realized that he shares many of the features enumerated in an attached checklist of "diagnostic" symptoms—especially a certain difficulty in concentrating and an easy irritability—and now wants what he himself calls "the stimulant that heals."

In response, I gamely point out a number of possible countervailing factors: that he may be taking a one-sided view of things, emphasizing his blemishes and overlooking his assets; that what he has already accomplished in his young life is inconsistent with attention deficit disorder; that many other reasons could be adduced for irritability and inattention; that Ritalin is an addictive substance. But in saying all this, I realize that I have also entered into a delicate negotiation, one that may end with his marching angrily from my office. For not only am I not doing what he wants, I am being insensitive, or so he will claim, to what "his" diagnosis clearly reveals. Less a suffering patient, he has been transformed, before my very eyes, into a dissatisfied customer.

It is a strange experience. People normally do not like to hear that they have a disease, but with this patient, as with many others like him, the opposite is the case: the conviction that he suffers from a mental disorder has somehow served to encourage him. On the one hand, it has rendered his life more interesting. On the other hand, it plays to the widespread current belief that everything can be made right with a pill. This pill will turn my young man into someone stronger, more in charge, less vulnerable—less ignoble. He wants it; it's for sale; end of discussion.

He is, as I say, hardly alone. With help from the popular media, home-brewed psychiatric diagnoses have proliferated in recent years, preoccupying the worried imaginations of the American public. Restless, impatient people are convinced that they have attention deficit disorder (ADD); anxious, vigilant people that they suffer from post-traumatic stress disorder (PTSD); stubborn, orderly, perfectionistic people that they are afflicted with obsessive-compulsive disorder (OCD); shy, sensitive people that they manifest avoidant personality disorder (APD), or social phobia. All have been persuaded that what are really matters of their individuality are, instead, medical problems and as such are to be solved with drugs. Those drugs will relieve the features of temperament that are burdensome, replacing them with features that please. The motto of this movement (with apologies to the DuPont corporation) might be "Better living through pharmacology."

And—most worrisome of all—wherever they look, such people find psychiatrists willing, even eager, to accommodate them. Worse, in many cases, it is psychiatrists who are leading the charge. But the exact role of the psychiatric profession in our current proliferation of disorders and in the thoughtless prescription of medication for them is no simple tale to tell.

When it comes to diagnosing mental disorders, psychiatry has undergone a sea change over the past two decades. The stages of that change can be traced in successive editions of the *Diagnostic and Statistical Manual of Mental Disorders* (DSM), the official tome of American psychiatry published and promoted by the American Psychiatric Association (APA). But historically its impetus derives—inadvertently—from a salutary effort begun in the early 1970s at the medical school of Washington University in St. Louis to redress the dearth of research in American psychiatry.

The St. Louis scholars were looking into a limited number of well-established disorders. Among them was schizophrenia, an affliction that can manifest itself in diverse ways. What the investigators were striving for was to isolate clear and distinct symptoms that separated indubitable cases of schizophrenia from less certain ones. By creating a set of such "research diagnostic criteria," their hope was to permit study to proceed across and among laboratories, free of the concern that erroneous conclusions might arise from the investigation of different types of patients in different medical centers.

With these criteria, the St. Louis group did not claim to have found the specific *features* of schizophrenia—a matter, scientifically speaking, of "validity." Rather, they were identifying certain markers or signs that would enable comparative study of the disease at multiple research sites—a matter of "reliability." But this very useful effort had baleful consequences when, in planning DSM-III (1980), the third edition of its *Diagnostic and Statistical Manual,* the APA picked up on the need for reliability and out of it forged a bid for scientific validity. In both DSM-III and DSM-IV (1994), what had been developed at St. Louis as a tool of scholarly research into only a few established disorders became subtly transformed, emerging as a clinical method of diagnosis (and, presumably, treatment) of psychiatric states and conditions of all kinds, across the board. The signs and markers—the presenting symptoms—became the official guide to the identification of mental disorders, and the list of such disorders served in turn to certify their existence in categorical form.

The significance of this turn to classifying mental disorders by their appearances cannot be underestimated. In physical medicine, doctors have long been aware that appearances, either as the identifying marks of disorder or as the targets of therapy, are untrustworthy. For one thing, it is sometimes difficult to distinguish symptoms of illness from normal variations in human life. For another, identical symptoms can be the products of totally different causal mechanisms and thus call for quite different treatments. For still another, descriptions of appearances are limitless, as limitless as the number of individuals presenting them; if medical classifications were to be built upon such descriptions, the enumerating of diseases would never end.

For all these reasons, general medicine abandoned appearance-based classifications more than a century ago. Instead, the signs and symptoms manifested by a given patient are understood to be produced by one or another underlying pathological process. Standard medical and surgical conditions are now categorized according to seven such processes: infectious disorders, neoplastic disorders, cardiovascular disorders, toxic/traumatic disorders, autoimmune disorders, genetic/degenerative disorders, and endocrine/metabolic disorders. Internists are reluctant to accept the existence of any proposed new disease unless its signs and symptoms can be linked to one of these processes.

The medical advances made possible by this approach can be appreciated by considering gangrene. Early in the nineteenth century, doctors differentiated between two types of this condition: "wet" and "dry." If a doctor was confronted with a gangrene that appeared wet, he or she was enjoined to dry it; if dry, to moisten it. Today, by contrast, doctors distinguish gangrenes of infection from gangrenes of arterial obstruction/infarction and treat each accordingly. The results, since they are based solidly in biology, are commensurately successful.

In DSM-led psychiatry, however, this beneficial movement has been forgone: today, psychiatric conditions are routinely differentiated by appearances alone. This means that the decision to follow a particular course of treatment for, say, depression is typically based not on the neurobiological or psychological data but on the presence or absence of certain associated symptoms like anxiety—that is, on the "wetness" or "dryness" of the depressive patient.

No less unsettling is the actual means by which mental disorders and their qualifying symptoms have come to find their way onto the lists in DSM-III and -IV. In the absence of validating conceptions like the seven mechanisms of disease in internal medicine, American psychiatry has turned to "committees of experts" to define mental disorder. Membership on such committees is a matter of one's reputation in the APA—which means that those chosen can confidently be expected to manifest not only a requisite degree of psychiatric competence but, perhaps more crucial, some talent for diplomacy and self-promotion.

In identifying psychiatric disorders and their symptoms, these "experts" draw upon their clinical experience and presuppositions. True, they also turn to the professional literature, but this literature is far from dependable or even stable. Much of it partakes of what the psychiatrist-philosopher Karl Jaspers once termed "efforts of Sisyphus": what was thought to be true today is often revealed to be false tomorrow. As a result, the final decisions by the experts on what constitutes a psychiatric condition and which symptoms define it rely excessively on the prejudices of the day.

Nor are the experts disinterested parties in these decisions. Some—

because of their position as experts—receive extravagant annual retainers from pharmaceutical companies that profit from the promotion of disorders treatable by the company's medications. Other venal interests may also be at work: when a condition like attention deficit disorder or multiple personality disorder appears in the official catalog of diagnoses, its treatment can be reimbursed by insurance companies, thus bringing direct financial benefit to an expert running a so-called trauma center or multiple personality unit. Finally, there is the inevitable political maneuvering within committees as one expert supports a second's opinion on a particular disorder with the tacit understanding of reciprocity when needed.

The new DSM approach of using experts and descriptive criteria in identifying psychiatric diseases has encouraged a productive industry. If you can describe it, you can name it; and if you can name it, then you can claim that it exists as a distinct "entity" with, eventually, a direct treatment tied to it. Proposals for new psychiatric disorders have multiplied so feverishly that the DSM itself has grown from a mere 119 pages in 1968 to 886 pages in the latest edition; a new and enlarged edition, DSM-V, is already in the planning stages. Embedded within these hundreds of pages are some categories of disorders that are real; some that are dubious, in the sense that they are more like the normal responses of sensitive people than psychiatric "entities"; and some that are purely the inventions of their proponents.

Let us get down to cases. The first clear example of the new approach at work occurred in the late 1970s, when a coalition of psychiatrists in the Veterans Administration (VA) and advocates for Vietnam War veterans propelled a condition called chronic post-traumatic stress disorder (PTSD) into DSM-III. It was, indeed, a perfect choice— itself a traumatic product, one might say, of the Vietnam War and all the conflicts and guilts that experience engendered—and it opened the door of the DSM to other and later disorders.

Emotional distress during and after combat (and other traumatic events) has been recognized since the mid-nineteenth century. The symptoms of "shell shock," as it came to be known in World War I, consist of a lingering anxiety, a tendency toward nightmares, "flashback memories" of battle, and the avoidance of activities that might provoke a sensation of danger. What was added after Vietnam was the belief that—perhaps because of a physical brain change due to the stress of combat—veterans who were not properly treated could become chronically disabled. This lifelong disablement would explain, in turn, such other problems as family disruption, unemployment, or alcohol and drug abuse.

Once the concept of a chronic form of PTSD with serious complications was established in DSM-III, patients claiming to have it crowded into VA hospitals. A natural alliance formed between patients and doctors to certify the existence of the disorder: patients received the privileges of the sick, while doctors received steady employment at a time when, with the end of the conflict in Southeast Asia, hospital beds were emptying. Anyone expressing skepticism about the validity of PTSD as a psychiatric condition—on the ground, say, that it had become a catchall category for people with long-standing disorders of temperament or behavior who were sometimes seeking to shelter themselves from responsibility—was dismissed as hostile to veterans or ignorant of the mental effects of fearful experiences.

Lately, however, the pro-PTSD forces have come under challenge in a major study that followed a group of Vietnam veterans through their treatment at the Yale-affiliated VA hospital in West Haven, Connecticut, and afterward. The participants in the study had received medications, group and individual therapy, behavioral therapy, family therapy, and vocational guidance—all concentrating on PTSD symptoms and the war experiences that had allegedly generated them. Upon discharge from the hospital, these patients did report some improvement in their drug and family problems, as well as a greater degree of hopefulness and self-esteem. Yet, within a mere eighteen months, their psychiatric symptoms, family problems, and personal relationships had actually become worse than on admission. They had made more suicide attempts, and their drug and alcohol abuse continued unabated. In short, prolonged and intensive hospital treatment for chronic PTSD had had no long-term beneficial effects whatsoever on the veterans' symptoms.

This report, which brings into doubt not only the treatment but the nature of the underlying "disease," has produced many agonized debates within the VA. Enthusiasts for PTSD argue that the investigators somehow missed the patients' "real" states of mind while at the same time overlooking subtle but nonetheless positive responses to treatment. They have also stepped up the search for biological evidence of brain changes produced by the emotional trauma of combat—changes that might validate chronic PTSD as a distinct condition and justify characterizing certain patients as its victims regardless of whether a successful treatment yet exists for it. In the psychiatric journals, reports of such a "biological marker" come and go.

Yet while we await final word on chronic PTSD, the skeptics—both within and without the VA system—would appear to hold much the stronger hand. They have pointed, for example, to analogous research on war veterans in Israel. According to Israeli psychiatrists, long-term treatment in hospitals has the unfortunate tendency of making battle-trauma victims hypersensitive to their symptoms and, by encouraging them to concentrate on the psychological wounds of combat, distracts their attention from the "here-and-now" problems of adjusting to peacetime demands and responsibilities.

This makes sense. After any traumatic event—whether we are speaking of a minor automobile accident, combat in war, or a civilian disaster like the Coconut Grove fire in Boston in 1942—exposed individuals will undergo a disquieted, disturbed state of mind that takes time to dissipate, depending on (among other things) the severity of the event and the temperament of the victim. As with grief, these mental states are natural—indeed, "built-in," species-specific—emotional responses. Customarily, they wane over time, leaving behind scars in the form of occasional dreams and nightmares but little more.

When a patient's reaction does not follow this standard course, one need hardly leap to conclude he or she is suffering from an "abnormal" or "chronic" or "delayed" form of PTSD. More likely, the culprit will be a separate and complicating condition like (most commonly) major depression, with its cardinal symptoms of misery, despair, and self-recrimination. In this condition, memories of past losses, defeats, or traumas are reawakened, giving content and justification to diminished attitudes about oneself. But such memories should hardly be confused with the cause of the depression itself, which can and should be treated for what it is. America's war veterans, who are entitled to our respect and support, surely deserve better than to be maintained in a state of chronic invalidism.

Medical errors characteristically assume three forms: oversimplification, misplaced emphasis, and invention. When it comes to chronic PTSD, all three were committed. Explanation of symptoms were oversimplified, with combat experiences being given priority quite apart from such factors as long-standing personality disorders, independent (post-combat) psychiatric conditions including major depression, or chronic psychological invalidism produced by prolonged hospitalization. Misplaced emphasis followed oversimplification when treatment concentrated on the psychological wounds of combat to the neglect of here-and-now problems that many patients were dodging, overlooking, or minimizing. Finally, the inventive construction of a condition called chronic PTSD justified a broad network of service-related psychiatric centers devoted to maintaining the veterans in treatment whether or not they were getting better—and, as we have seen, they were not.

Variants of these same mistakes can be discerned in the identification and treatment of other diseases du jour. Multiple personality disorder (MPD), for example, posits an unconscious psychological mechanism, termed dissociation, that occurs in people facing a traumatic life event. When such dissociation occurs, it disrupts the integrative action of consciousness, causing patients to fail to link experience with memory.

Typical dissociative "conditions" include dissociative amnesia, dissociative fugues, and dissociative identity disorder, the last named being the DSM-IV term for MPD. Thus, a person who leaves home and travels to another city only to remember nothing of the interval and amazed to find him- or herself away from home is said to have undergone a state of dissociative fugue. Patients claiming they cannot recall prominent events—their school years, their childhood friends—are said to suffer from dissociative amnesia. Finally, a person who displays over time two or more personality states that take control of his or her behavior is said to be in a condition of dissociative identity disorder.

The problem with dissociation, as with so many purported unconscious mental processes, is that it cannot be discerned and studied apart from the behaviors it is intended to explain. What generates and sustains those behaviors is the power of their effect on others, whether doctors or onlookers. But once attention has been transferred from the behavior itself to the imagined mental state of the patient exhibiting it, a diagnosis—dissociation—can be triumphantly invoked through reasoning that goes in circles: Why don't I remember first grade?/Because you have dissociated your memory./How do

you know that?/Because you can't remember first grade. This justifies, in turn, a long, arcane, melodramatic process of treatment.

MPD is, in fact, a form of hysteria—that is, a behavior that *mimics*
physical or psychiatric disorder. Hysteria often takes the form of
complaints of affliction or displays of dysfunction by people who have
been led to believe that they are sick. More than occasionally, those
doing the leading are the psychiatrists themselves, especially those in
the business of helping patients recover "repressed" or "dissociated"
memories of childhood sexual abuse.

It was the 1973 best-selling book (and later TV movie) *Sybil*,
describing an abused patient with sixteen personalities, that launched
the whole copycat epidemic of MPD. That book has recently been
unmasked as a fraud. According to Dr. Herbert Spiegel of Columbia
University, who knew the patient in question and disputed her case
with the author of the book prior to its publication, Sybil was in
fact "a wonderful hysterical patient with role confusion, which is
typical of high hysterics." Spiegel, whose protests at the time got him
nowhere—"If we don't call it a multiple personality, we don't have a
book! The publishers want it to be that, otherwise it won't sell!" he
quotes the author as remonstrating—observes ruefully that "this
chapter . . . will go down in history as an embarrassing phase of
American psychiatry."▲

Although the MPD epidemic is now subsiding, the "disease" itself
remains enshrined in DSM-III and DSM-IV, a textbook case of an
alleged disorder whose identification is based entirely on appearances and then sustained as valid by its listing in DSM. So it is, too,
with adult attention deficit disorder and social phobia.

Defined as a tendency to fear embarrassment in situations where
one is exposed to scrutiny by others, social phobia relates in about 90
percent of cases to a fear of public speaking, an almost universal
condition that can usually be overcome by practice. Some psychiatrists claim that one of eight Americans suffers from this supposed
disorder and should receive pharmacological treatment for it. If that
figure were accurate, we would be confronted with a mental disorder

▲The role of the "repressed-memory" movement in a whole line of celebrated cases
and legal trials, from supposed satanic rituals to the alleged sexual abuse of children in
schools and day-care centers, is a subject unto itself. I have reviewed this issue in
"Psychotherapy Awry," *American Scholar*, Winter 1994.

CST - "Common Sense Therapy" - Dr. Nabokin

almost as common as depression and alcoholism—a dubious proposition on its face. Whether medication to make patients more comfortable (but perhaps less self-critical) in their public speaking will improve their lives or careers is another question altogether.

As for ADD, a diagnosis of that condition often rests on a perceived failure to attend to details: mistakes are made, and work performance is impaired, by restlessness and difficulty in concentrating. This, too, is a characteristic of many people, one that can emerge with particular salience in the face of challenges at home or work or with the onset of an illness like depression or mania. An individual seeking treatment for it may be expressing nothing more than a desire for "self-improvement." Whether it is the proper role of a prescription-dispensing psychiatrist to act as the patient's agent in such an enterprise is, again, another question altogether.

Although people may differ in such qualities as attentiveness and confidence, it is simply not true that most individuals deficient in these qualities are sick. What *is* true is that they will be changed by the medications proposed to heal the alleged sickness. Everyone is more attentive when on Ritalin; many are less emotionally responsive when on selective serotonin reuptake inhibitors (SSRIs) like Prozac or Paxil. That emotional and cognitive changes are associated with certain drugs should come as no surprise—even small amounts of alcohol will loosen one's inhibitions. But that hardly means that the inhibitions constitute a mental disorder.

For the psychiatrists involved, there is another consideration here. In colluding with their patients' desire for self-improvement, they implicitly enter a claim to know what the ideal human temperament should be, toward which they make their various pharmacological adjustments and manipulations. On this point, Thomas Szasz, the vociferous critic of psychiatry, is right: such exercises in mental cosmetics should be offensive to anyone who values the richness of human psychological diversity. Both medically and morally, encumbering this naturally occurring diversity with the terminology of disease is a first step toward efforts, however camouflaged, to control it.

Why are psychiatrists not more like other doctors—differentiating patients by the causes of their illnesses and offering treatments specifically linked to the mechanisms of these illnesses? One reason is that they cannot be. In contrast to cardiologists, dermatologists, ophthalmologists, and other medical practitioners, physicians who study and treat disorders of mind and behavior are unable to demonstrate how symptoms emerge directly from activity in, or changes to, the organ that generates them—namely, the brain. Indeed, many of the profession's troubles, especially the false starts and misdirections that have plagued it from the beginning, stem from the mind/brain problem, the most critical issue in the natural sciences and a fundamental obstacle to all students of consciousness.

It was because of the mind/brain problem that Sigmund Freud, wedded as he was to an explanatory rather than a descriptive approach in psychiatry, decided to delineate causes for mental disorders that implicitly presupposed brain mechanisms (while not depending on an explicit knowledge of such mechanisms). In brief, Freud's "explanation" evoked a conflict between, on the one hand, brain-generated drives (which could be identified by their psychological manifestations) and, on the other hand, socially imposed prohibitions on the expression and satisfaction of those same drives. This conflict was believed to produce a "dynamic unconscious" when mental and behavioral abnormalities emerged.

This explanation had its virtues and seemed to help "ordinary" people reacting to life's troubles in an understandable way. But it was not suited to the *seriously* mentally ill—schizophrenics and manic-depressives, for example—who did not respond to explanation-based treatments. That is one of the factors that by the 1970s, when it became overwhelmingly clear that such people did respond satisfactorily to physical treatments and, especially, to medication, impelled the move away from hypothetical explanations (as in Freud) to empirical descriptions of manifest symptoms (as in DSM-III and -IV). Another was the long-standing failure of American psychiatry, when guided by Freudian presumptions, to advance research, a failure that led, among other things, to the countervailing efforts of the investigators in St. Louis.

At first, indeed, the new descriptive approach seemed to represent significant progress, enhancing communication among psychiatrists, stimulating research, and holding out the promise of a new era of creative growth in psychiatry itself, a field grown stultified by its decades-long immersion in psychoanalytic theory. Today, however, twenty years after its imposition, the weaknesses inherent in a system of classification based on appearances—and contaminated by self-interested advocacy—have become glaringly evident.

In my own view, and despite the obstacles presented by the mind/brain problem, psychiatry need not abandon the path of medicine. Essentially, psychiatric disorders come under four large groupings (and their subdivisions), each of them distinguished causally from the other three and bearing a different relationship to the brain.

The first grouping comprises patients who have physical diseases or damage to the brain that can provoke psychiatric symptoms: these include patients with Alzheimer disease and schizophrenia. In the second grouping are those who are intermittently distressed by some aspect of their mental constitution—a weakness in their cognitive power or an instability in their affective control—when facing challenges in school, employment, or marriage. Unlike those in the first category, those in the second do not *have* disease or any obvious damage to the brain; rather, they are vulnerable because of who they *are*—that is, how they are constituted.

The third category consists of those whose behavior—alcoholism, drug addiction, sexual paraphilia, anorexia nervosa, and the like—has become a warped way of life. They are patients not because of what they have or who they are but because of what they are *doing* and how they have become conditioned to doing it. In the fourth category, finally, are those in need of psychiatric assistance because of emotional reactions provoked by events that injure or thwart their commitments, hopes, and aspirations. They suffer from states of mind like grief, homesickness, jealousy, demoralization—states that derive not from what they have or who they are or what they are doing but from what they have *encountered* in life.

Each of these distress-generating mechanisms will shape a different course of treatment, and its study should direct research in a unique direction. Thus, brain diseases are to be cured, alleviated, and prevented. Individuals with constitutional weaknesses need strengthening and guidance and perhaps, under certain stressful situations, medication for their emotional responses. Damaging behaviors need to be interrupted and patients troubled by them assisted in overcoming their appeal. Individuals suffering grief and demoralization need both understanding and redirection from circumstances that elicit or maintain such states of mind. Finally, for psychiatric patients who show several mechanisms in action simultaneously, a coordinated sequence of treatments is required.

But the details are not important. What is important is the general approach. Psychiatrists have for too long been satisfied with assessments of human problems that generate only a categorical diagnosis followed by a prescription for medication. Urgently required is a diagnostic and therapeutic formulation that can comprehend several interactive sources of disorder and sustain a complex program of treatment and rehabilitation. Until psychiatry begins to organize its observations, explanatory hypotheses, and therapeutics in such a coherent way, it will remain as entrapped in its present classificatory system as medicine was in the nineteenth century, unable to explain itself to patients, to their families, to the public—or even to itself.

That is not all. In its recent infatuation with symptomatic, push-button remedies, psychiatry has lost its way not only intellectually but spiritually and morally. Even when it is not actually doing damage to the people it is supposed to help, as in the case of veterans with chronic PTSD, it is encouraging among doctors and patients alike the fraudulent and dangerous fantasy that life's every passing "symptom" can be clinically diagnosed and, once diagnosed, alleviated, if not eliminated, by pharmacological intervention. This idea is as false to reality, and ultimately to human hopes, as it is destructive of everything the subtle and beneficial art of psychiatry has meant to accomplish.

Commentary, 1999

Romancing Depression

Of all the medical disciplines, psychiatry is the most closely tied to cultural attitudes. So it is hardly surprising that, along with our culture itself, American psychiatric thought and practice should have undergone radical change since the 1960s and 1970s. What may seem more surprising is that, at least in its later phases, this shift has followed not the surface fancies and leftist ideologies of the age but deeper currents of realism and pragmatism. Just as socialist politics and economies collapsed and were replaced by a newfound admiration for democratic capitalism, so dogmatic Freudianism, with its guilt-assuaging visions of intrapsychic conflict and its view that unconscious Oedipal anxiety explains all mental disorder, came to be replaced by more realistic assumptions and by empirical studies of mental illness and its treatment.

In particular, recent decades have seen two fundamental psychiatric upheavals: one in therapy, the other in the identification and treatment of two major mental illnesses, manic-depression and schizophrenia. Both upheavals, of which the first is the lesser known, ended up enhancing psychiatric practice and benefiting patients and their families.

By the end of the 1960s, a number of psychiatrists had already come to acknowledge that, in standard practice, psychotherapy tended to tolerate self-indulgent, aggressive, and impulsive behavior, in most cases explaining it away as a defense against anxiety. But this, it was becoming clear, worked against the recovery of patients, let alone their emotional maturation. What began to emerge in the 1970s was a more demanding psychotherapy, one in which patients were expected to bring their behavior under control before help could be found for their emotional distress.

The initial outlines of the new psychotherapy were most astutely articulated by the iconoclastic psychoanalyst Otto Kernberg of New York. In his concept of the "borderline" patient, Kernberg identified a large group of individuals showing a pervasive pattern of emotional and behavioral instability. Typically, their interpersonal relationships

60

were characterized by dramatic, often violent alternations between anger and affection. Intense displays of temper, angry separations from relatives and friends, even physical fighting were common, as were unpredictable mood shifts leading to chaotic sexual behavior.

Psychiatrists were well acquainted with patients like these, to whom they gave diagnostic names like pseudoneurotic schizophrenics or intense narcissistic personalities. Generally, they were thought to be inaccessible to therapy. Kernberg, however, focused not on their personalities but on their conduct. Even in the therapeutic setting itself, he observed, such patients would manipulate and polarize, set up false dichotomies (as between presumptive "friends" and "enemies"), and thereby excuse their own often inexcusable behavior. This, said Kernberg, had to be countered. If there was to be any chance of helping these people, they needed to be taken to task and held accountable.

Liberating therapists from their own self-imposed shackles of permissiveness, Kernberg encouraged them to confront aggressive and narcissistic patients who had previously defeated them and force these patients to take responsibility for their feelings and behavior. And indeed, the application of Kernberg's ideas did bring into therapeutic care many individuals previously excluded from attention, in the process helping them overcome the attitudes that had previously crippled them. Kernberg's ideas soon spread beyond the specific class of patients he had identified to include other people in other circumstances who suffered from similar tendencies.

In the meantime, and alongside these improvements in the capacities of psychotherapists, an entirely different idea was emerging: namely, that many of the seriously mentally ill—specifically, those suffering from manic-depression and schizophrenia—were not simply expressing deep-seated psychological conflicts, as Freudianism had taught, but had real, *medical* diseases. Prompting this conceptual breakthrough was the chance discovery in those years of medications like lithium, which both corrected specific conditions and relieved patients of other symptoms that had proved resistant to psychiatric treatment.

Over the ensuing decades, much has been written about this second development, including by patients or former patients who in describing their own ordeals have placed the advances of psychiatry in the light of personal experience. One such patient is the writer Andrew Solomon, whose book *The Noonday Demon: An Atlas of Depression* caused a considerable stir when it was published earlier this year and has recently been nominated for a National Book Award. *The Noonday Demon* joins such other accounts of depression as *Darkness Visible* (1990) by the novelist William Styron and *An Unquiet Mind* (1995) by Kay Redfield Jamison, a well-known academic psychologist, but it is much more ambitious in scope. Inadvertently, it also reveals how many of the temperaments and attitudes challenged by Otto Kernberg continue to linger—and to be indulged.

As his subtitle implies, Solomon means to do more than describe for us his own life and his encounter with depressive illness—though he certainly does that in very great detail. He also set out to characterize the entire state of current professional thinking about depression, the vast array of therapies applied to it around the world, and the history and politics of its study. All of this is undoubtedly of interest, if marred by Solomon's fundamentally uncritical attitude toward the information he has assembled and his tendency to see benefit in every treatment he encounters.

Over the course of this book we certainly learn much about Andrew Solomon. He is independently wealthy—his father directs a profitable pharmaceutical company that produces, mirabile dictu, an antidepressant. He is well educated, with an M.A. from an English university, has written for the *New Yorker*, and conducts an active social life. Also, he is sexually adventurous, choosing both female and male partners. And he has tried a wide variety of addictive drugs, although he claims that he never became dependent on any of them because he lacks, as he puts it, "an addictive personality."

As for his depression, the first attacks, Solomon says, seemed to come out of the blue and at a time when he thought he had "solved most of [his] problems." As the depression worsened, all his emotions turned downward, he found it progressively harder to find joy in anything, and ultimately he withdrew to his bed, stopped eating, and fell into a stuporous, self-neglectful condition from which he was rescued, essentially, by his father.

There followed many different kinds and forms of treatment, including but hardly limited to both orthodox psychoanalysis and pharmacological medication. With the help of the latter, Solomon recovered from his initial spell of depression, but in the next few years he fell into two more, almost as severe, both of which were precipitated by physical illness and the cessation of medication. In each case he was beset by self-loathing, became preoccupied with thoughts of death, and engaged in the crudest forms of sexual behavior in order to expose himself to HIV and thus gain a real excuse for suicide. Nothing he could do or think about would relieve his symptoms. In the end, only working out an efficacious regimen of pills has helped him and kept him well.

We learn all about Solomon's many treatments in this book and also about the problems each type entailed. As he became more and more convinced of the biomedical nature of his condition, he studied the theories behind antidepressant medications and the way they act on different patients, and this research, too, he shares in detail with his readers. He also visited many different psychiatric centers and healing places, from the conventional to the outré, inquiring in each case into patients who experienced states of mind similar to his own and the way therapists and physicians responded to these patients and what advances they anticipated in knowledge and methods of practice. The record of all these experiences—along with interviews of leaders of the psychiatric profession and a broad review of the contemporary periodical literature—fills out the book.

Aside from the many things we learn about the adventures of Andrew Solomon, however, what exactly do we learn about depression? To answer that question it is useful to compare *The Noonday Demon* with the memoirs by William Styron and Kay Redfield Jamison. They, too, describe from a personal viewpoint the mental changes wrought by depression and mania and offer detailed accounts of treatment, particularly by means of drugs and electric shock. Both authors are exceptionally good at portraying the loss of control felt during attacks of depression, especially the irrational but all-encompassing despair that accompanies it. Thus, Styron at one point compares his depressed mind to "one of those outmoded small-town telephone exchanges, being gradually inundated by flood-waters," while for Jamison the engulfing sense of personal worthlessness and hopelessness made her regard even her body as "uninhabitable . . . raging and weeping and full of destruction."

The precision with which these writers strive to capture the stages of their condition, from onset to eventual recovery, marks something of a contrast with Solomon's often blurry reportage and omnium-gatherum approach to medical information. More important, both of them bring into focus, as he does not, the particular *form* of depression that all three suffered from. For, as a mental symptom, depression can have many different causes and can also manifest itself in an entire range of feelings, from discouragement and demoralization to something much more elemental. The depression that these books are describing—here again Solomon's approach tends to muddle necessary distinctions—is of the latter variety.

To be still more precise, this form of depression is a symptom or, better, an expression of what is called affective disorder. This is an affliction in which an otherwise ordinary mental faculty—namely, the link between the mind's affective domain (moods, emotions, and drives) and the mind's cognitive domain (thoughts and perceptions)—has been disrupted. As a consequence, affects run autonomously and ungoverned, shifting with any given attack of the disorder either toward the misery and withdrawal of depression or toward the energy and overconfidence of mania. That is why most psychiatrists prefer to use more exact terms like *manic-depression* or *bipolar disorder* to refer to this class of affective illnesses, although for ease of understanding I shall continue to refer to it by the somewhat misleading catchall *depression*.

Many people, including many patients, still believe that at the heart of this particular disorder lies some great personal and moral flaw, one that can be corrected if only they would not let their emotions run amok. The great virtue of the Styron and Jamison books, especially if read in conjunction with more specialized studies like Francis M. Mondimore's *Depression, the Mood Disease* (1990), is that they help dispel this mistaken notion. Rather, they demonstrate, this form of depression shares more attributes with a disease like epilepsy than it does with a character trait like self-pity—and, like epilepsy, it can respond to medical treatment. Kay Jamison, in particular, has inspired many victims of depression to realize that if they can overcome this mental ordeal as she did, they might at last put it behind them and move on into life.

Andrew Solomon's book is much more equivocal in its message. Although thorough to a fault as a description of personal experience, and no less exhaustive in its account of treatments and the theoretical conceptions behind them, it is, at its heart, a book about *him* and correspondingly less than useful either as a true "atlas" of depression or as a guide for fellow sufferers.

The problem comes to light right at the start, with Solomon's portentous first sentence: "Depression is the flaw in love." Similar aphoristic statements turn up again and again: "Depression like sex retains an unquenchable aura of mystery. It is new every time." "Strength of will is the best bulwark against depression." Not only are these assertions melodramatic, they are quite simply—and revealingly—wrong.

To repeat, the particular disorder at issue here is a disease, an affliction that disrupts a natural function of emotional control. This disease, like other diseases both physical and mental, renders the afflicted person impaired in ways that are *essentially the same from case to case.* The injury is no more related to "love" than it is to any other emotion: *all* affective functions are disrupted. And far from being "new every time," it is so similar from occasion to occasion that a veteran patient—or an experienced relative—can detect its recurrence from the first subtle effects on emotional tone, attitude, facial expression, even posture. Finally, strength of will has no more to do with this disorder and its course than strength of will controls the progress of Alzheimer disease.

The awful but crucial thing about disease, mental or physical, is that it stands apart from who you are as a person. *You* can be discouraged, demoralized, and downhearted about events in your life that have blocked your hopes and plans. If you happen to be selfish, willful, and irresponsible, you might drive others away and thus bring on symptoms of loneliness and despair. If you take up attitudes and assumptions that promote anorexia nervosa, alcoholism, or drug addiction, you might suffer the miseries these behaviors carry with them. These states of mind are often and confusingly labeled depression, but none of them is the depression I am talking about, which is not a *you* but an *it*, a thing unto itself and not just the dark side of human emotion.

You cannot choose for or against this disease. It chooses you, just as does epilepsy, cancer, or heart disease. It turns you into a stereotyped copy of every other person afflicted with it. You are not in charge of it, you are not to blame for it, and you can do little about it except to seek the help that may enable you to escape its clutches.

Styron and Jamison understand this. By contrast, Solomon seems in thrall to an earlier, quite romantic, and quite literary notion of mental illness. Although he stipulates that his first attack seems to have come out of nowhere, he also clearly regards it as emerging from deep within his psyche, as reflecting some intimate flaw that he has yet to work through. He is enamored of himself for *having* this flaw, and he is enamored of himself in the end for having worked through it. Along the way, he is even a little enamored of his behavior in the course of suffering it.

In one scene of this book, Solomon describes, and excuses, a vicious assault on one of his homosexual partners in which he broke the man's nose and jaw and sent him to the hospital in need of blood transfusions. Some of the physical sensations he felt as he delivered his bone-crushing blows were, he freely admits, pleasurable. More: even today, "part of me does not rue what happened, because I sincerely believe that [without it] I would have gone irretrievably crazy." And a bit later he adds: "Engaging in violent acts is not a good way to treat depression. It is, however, effective. To deny the inbred curative power of violence would be a terrible mistake."

At least one admiring reviewer of *The Noonday Demon* paused to point out that these statements might appear to justify acts that were, well, criminal. They certainly do that, not to mention that they conjure up images of brownshirt thuggery. But they also happen to flow naturally from Solomon's conception of depression less as an illness than as a stage on which to enact a heroic drama of the self.

So, too, does another picturesque scene in *The Noonday Demon* in which our hero undergoes an African ceremony called "ndeup": an "animist ritual that probably antedates voodoo" and that amounts to a kind of exorcism. On the recommendation of "the mother of a friend of the girlfriend of a friend," Solomon traveled to Senegal to undergo this treatment. There he was taken in hand by a mysterious priestess who supervised the ceremony. While he danced to drums being beaten by members of the local community, Solomon was smeared "on every inch" of his body with blood from a cockerel and a ram. The blood, caking like a scab, attracted thousands of flies. Five women dressed in loose-fitting robes and wearing belts filled with prayers and iconic objects danced about him as he chanted to his bewitching spirits, "Leave me be; give me peace; and let me do the work of my life. I will never forget you." The ceremony ended with a great barbecue of the ram.

Solomon does not say whether the treatment actually helped him, though he does allow that it "jolted the system, which could certainly throw one's brain chemistry into overdrive—a kind of unplugged ECT [electroconvulsive therapy]." It would be hard to argue with *that*.

Please do not misunderstand me. In depression, just as in any illness, including cardiac disease and cancer, *you* and *it* do exist together. You do not cause or control the disease, but you may make the expression of it stronger or weaker, the treatment of it easier or harder. This is a very important point and one that cannot be emphasized enough. But what *The Noonday Demon* gives us is a different and in many ways opposite scenario: a lonely existential fight against darkness and despair in which a star is born, whose name is Andrew. Romanticizing the *it*, Solomon is obtuse about the *you*, to the point of embracing acts of criminal violence as conducive to "sanity."

And this brings me back to Otto Kernberg and to the other revolution in the understanding of mental illness with which I began. Although Andrew Solomon managed not to encounter one, a growing number of psychotherapists these days are less willing to sit by as patients make up their own rules for living or disregard consequences and moral meanings. To the contrary, they tend to insist that patients take note of their own selfish attitudes and behaviors and recognize their role in generating the distress for which they seek treatment. In fact, one of the most difficult clinical problems today is figuring out how to differentiate disorders tied to a *you*, where therapeutic guidance and strengthening are essential, from the several *its* that damage mental faculties, are to be apprehended as diseases, and need to be cured and prevented.

The disciplines that surround psychiatry—neuroscience, psychology, pharmacology, and epidemiology—have brightened the prospects of dealing successfully with the particular affective disorder I have been calling depression. At the same time, the "judgmental" turn taken by psychotherapy has helped many a patient escape the trap of narcissism and emotional instability. To anyone who has followed or participated in the frequently destructive wars of the psychiatric profession, it cannot but be heartening that the recent turn to the pragmatic in therapy should be accompanied, and strengthened, by an essentially moral vision of human responsibility. The model celebrated by Andrew Solomon is, one earnestly prays, a throwback.

Commentary, 2001

Part II

THE PHYSICIAN-ASSISTED-SUICIDE DEBACLE

Physician-assisted suicide emerged most unexpectedly during my tenure as psychiatrist-in-chief at Hopkins and turned on matters of practice and understanding of medicine that had lain dormant since World War II. But it emerged with a vengeance and with a particular champion, Dr. Jack Kevorkian. What struck me was the epidemic-like spread of this idea—in its "anatomy" and not just in its momentum.

Epidemiologists recognize a triadic "anatomy" to epidemics, pointing out that one can identify "hosts," "agents," and "environment" as enmeshed causal factors starting and sustaining them. They also teach that recognizing these distinct but interrelated elements helps direct efforts at terminating an epidemic and preventing its recurrence.

By "hosts" the epidemiologists mean those victimized by the epidemic usually because of some vulnerability or lack of immunity to it. By "agents" they mean those processes or factors that damage or hurt the "hosts" (they may distinguish as "vectors" such carriers as mosquitoes or contaminated water supplies that carry the infectious bacterium or virus that is the actual agent). By "environment" they mean all the physical, social, and cultural aspects of life in which the hosts and agents exist and which can be easily overlooked in their provocative or sustaining roles in an epidemic.

I held that a convergence of interacting psychosocial factors embracing host, agent, and environment explained the outbreak of deaths from physician-assisted suicide in America. Vulnerable "hosts" (mentally disturbed by a variety of illnesses or suspected illnesses) living in an unprotecting "environment" (the social and judicial climate of contemporary American life) were lured to death by a provocative "vector/agent" (Jack Kevorkian and others who promoted the idea that doctors could often best help their patients by killing them). I saw the "hosts" as psychiatric patients, the "agents" as ideologues taking advantage of the hosts' mental vulnerabilities, and the "environment" as unwittingly supporting a sensibility that needed to be challenged. All three factors were important, but their convergence and interaction at this time strengthened each of them synergistically and gave momentum to the epidemic.

Fighting the Kevorkian epidemic drew my attention to the ceremonial rites at medical school graduations today. The oaths taken by the newly minted doctors displayed a remarkable commitment to subjectivity—to feelings and impulses—and this commitment far outtrumped any commitment to discerning the facts about the plight of the sick. The oaths specifically downplayed the need for medical experience and education to enhance the strenuous virtues of stamina, persistence, selflessness, and devotion to duty by which the professional mind learns to rule the body. "Romantic man" was proclaiming that feelings derived from experience rather than knowledge gave sanction to actions that were more protective of the doctors' "wellbeing" than that of the patients. As Jack Kevorkian demonstrates, doctors with such ideas are dangerous.

Finally I was drawn to look at the remarkable best-seller Tuesdays with Morrie *(1997) by Mitch Albom, expecting to find support for my views given that the author describes the heroic struggles of Morrie Schwartz with Lou Gehrig disease, amyotrophic lateral sclerosis. Although impressed by both the devotion of the author to his teacher and the teacher's coherent acceptance of his mortality, I was struck by a lack of general purpose behind this example. Its support for a kind of hedonistic nihilism weakened it as a weapon to fight the Kevorkian epidemic. My friend, the brilliant writer Joseph Epstein, suggested that I might entitle my essay "Tuesdays with Morrie, Wednesdays with Jack." We couldn't persuade the editor.*

The Kevorkian Epidemic

Dr. Jack Kevorkian of Detroit has been in the papers most days this past summer and autumn helping sick people kill themselves. He is said to receive hundreds of calls a week. Although his acts are illegal by statute and common law in Michigan, no one stops him. Many citizens, including members of three juries, believe he means well, perhaps thinking: Who knows? Just maybe, we ourselves shall need his services someday.

To me it looks like madness from every quarter. The patients are mad by definition in that they are suicidally depressed and demoralized; Dr. Kevorkian is "certifiable" in that his passions render him, as the state code specifies, "dangerous to others"; and the usually reliable people of Michigan are confused and anxious to the point of incoherence by terrors of choice that are everyday issues for doctors. These three disordered parties have converged, provoking a local epidemic of premature death.

Let me begin with the injured hosts of this epidemic, the patients mad by definition. At this writing, more than forty, as best we know, have submitted to Dr. Kevorkian's deadly charms. They came to him with a variety of medical conditions: Alzheimer disease, multiple sclerosis, chronic pain, amyotrophic lateral sclerosis, cancer, drug addiction, and more. These are certainly disorders from which anyone might seek relief. But what kind of relief do patients with these conditions usually seek when they do not have a Dr. Kevorkian to extinguish their pain?

Both clinical experience and research on this question are extensive—and telling. A search for death does not accompany most terminal or progressive diseases. Pain-ridden patients customarily call doctors for remedies, not for termination of life. Physical incapacity, as with advanced arthritis, does not generate suicide. Even amyotrophic lateral sclerosis, or Lou Gehrig disease, a harrowing condition I shall describe presently, is not associated with increased suicide among its sufferers. Most doctors learn these facts as they help patients and their families burdened by these conditions.

But we don't have to rely solely upon the testimonies of experienced physicians. Recently cancer patients in New England were asked about their attitudes toward death. The investigators—apparently surprised to discover a will to live when they expected to find an urge to die—reported in the *Lancet* (vol. 347, 1996, pp. 1805–1810) two striking findings. First, cancer patients enduring pain were not inclined to want euthanasia or physician-assisted suicide. In fact, "patients actually experiencing pain were more likely to find euthanasia or physician-assisted suicide unacceptable." Second, those patients inclined toward suicide—whether in pain or not—were suffering from depression. As the investigators noted: "These data indicate a conflict between attitudes and possible practices related to euthanasia and physician-assisted suicide. These *interventions* were approved of for terminally ill patients with unremitting pain, but these are not the patients most likely to request such *interventions*. . . . There is *some* concern that with legislation of euthanasia or physician-assisted suicide non-psychiatric physicians, who generally have a poor ability to detect and treat depression, may allow life-ending *interventions* when treatment of depression may be more appropriate." (Italics added to identify mealymouthed expressions: *interventions* means homicides, and *some* means that we investigators should stay cool in our concerns—after all, it's not we who are dying.)

None of this is news to psychiatrists who have studied suicides associated with medical illnesses. Depression, the driving force in most cases, comes in two varieties: symptomatic depression found as a feature of particular diseases—that is, as one of the several symptoms of that disease; and demoralization, the common state of mind of people in need of guidance but facing discouraging circumstances alone. Both forms of depression render patients vulnerable to feelings of hopelessness that, if not adequately confronted, may lead to suicide.

Let me first concentrate on the symptomatic depressions because an understanding of them illuminates much of the problem. By the term *symptomatic*, psychiatrists mean that with some physical diseases suicidal depression is one of the condition's characteristic features. Careful students of these diseases come to appreciate that this variety of depression is not to be accepted as a natural feeling of discouragement provoked by bad circumstances—that is, similar to the down-hearted state of, say, a bankrupt man or a grief-stricken widow. Instead, the depression we are talking about here, with its beclouding of judgment, sense of misery, and suicidal inclinations, is a symptom identical in nature to the fevers, pains, or loss of energy that are signs of the disease itself.

A good and early example of the recognition of symptomatic depression is found in George Huntington's classical (1872) description of the disorder eventually named after him: Huntington disease. Huntington had first seen the condition when he was a youth visiting patients with his father, a family doctor on Long Island. He noted that one of the characteristic features of the condition was "the tendency to . . . that form of insanity which leads to suicide." Even now, between 7 and 10 pecent of nonhospitalized patients with Huntington disease do succeed in killing themselves. Psychiatrists and neurologists have perceived that Parkinson disease, multiple sclerosis, Alzheimer disease, AIDS dementia, and some cerebral-vascular strokes all have this same tendency to provoke "that form of insanity which leads to suicide."

That these patients are insane is certain. They are overcome with a sense of hopelessness and despair, often with the delusional belief that they are in some way useless, burdensome, or even corrupt perpetrators of evil. One of my patients with Huntington disease felt that Satan was dwelling within her and that she acted in accordance with his wishes. These patients lose their capacity to concentrate and reason; they have a pervasive and unremitting feeling of gloom and a constant, even eager willingness to accept death. These characteristics of symptomatic depression recur in all the diseases mentioned above. Multiple sclerosis (MS) patients are frequently afflicted by it. Some five or six of Dr. Kevorkian's patients had MS.

The problematic nature of symptomatic depression goes beyond the painful state of mind of the patient. Other observers—such as family members and physicians—may well take the depressive's disturbed, indeed insane, point of view as a proper assessment of his or her situation. It was this point that Huntington, long before the time of modern antidepressant treatment, wished to emphasize by identifying it as an insanity. He knew that failure to diagnose this feature will lead to the neglect of efforts to treat the patient properly and to protect him or her from suicide until the symptom remits.

Such neglect is a crucial blunder because, whether the underlying condition is Huntington disease, Alzheimer disease, MS, or something else, modern antidepressant treatment is usually effective at relieving the mood disorder and restoring the patient's emotional equilibrium. In Michigan and in Holland, where physician-assisted suicide also takes place, these actions to hasten death are the ultimate neglect of patients with symptomatic depression; they are, really, a form of collusion with insanity.

The diagnosis of symptomatic depression is not overly difficult if its existence is remembered and its features systematically sought. But many of its characteristics—such as its capacity to provoke bodily pains—are not known to all physicians. That such depression occurs in dire conditions, such as Huntington disease, may weigh against its prompt diagnosis and treatment. Again and again, kindly intended physicians presume that a depression "makes sense"—given the patient's situation—and overlook the stereotypical signs of the insanity. They presume justifiable demoralization and forget the pharmacologically treatable depressions.

Over the past decade, at least among psychiatrists, the reality of symptomatic depressions has become familiar, and treatment readiness has become the rule. Yet not all sick patients with life-threatening depression have symptomatic depressions. Many physically ill patients are depressed for perfectly understandable reasons, given the grueling circumstances of their progressive and intractable disease. Just as any misfortune can provoke grief and anxiety, so can awareness of loss of health and of a closed future.

Well titled *demoralization*, this depression, too, has a number of attributes. It waxes and wanes with experiences and events, comes in waves, and is worse at certain times—such as during the night, when contemplating future discomforts and burdens, and when the patient is alone or uninstructed about the benefits that modern treatments can bring him.

In contrast to the symptomatic depressions, which run their own course almost independent of events, demoralization is sensitive to circumstances and especially to the conduct of doctors toward the patient. Companionship, especially that which provides understanding and clear explanations of the actions to be taken in opposing disease and disability, can be immensely helpful in overcoming this state and sustaining the patient in a hopeful frame of mind.

The obverse is also true. If faced by inattentive physicians—absentee physicians most commonly—patients can become more discouraged and utterly demoralized by what they assume is their physician's resignation from a hopeless battle. All patients afflicted with disease—curable or incurable—are susceptible to bleak assumptions about their future and their value. These susceptibilities can be magnified or diminished by the behavior of their physicians.

The therapeutic implication here is that despairing assumptions wither if directly combated and shown to be an inaccurate analysis of the situation. Demoralization is an eminently treatable mental condition. Hopeless doctors, however, ready to see patients as untreatable, produce hopeless patients. The combination of the two produces a zeal for terminating effort. "What's the point?" becomes the cry of both patient and doctor. *Self-fulfilling prophecy*

This is the point: Depression, both in the form of a symptomatic mental state and in the form of demoralization, is the result of illness and circumstances combined and is treatable just as are other effects of illness. These treatments are the everyday skills of many physicians, but particularly of those physicians who are specialists in these disorders and can advance the treatments most confidently.

Most suicidally depressed patients are not rational individuals who have weighed the balance sheet of their lives and discovered more red than black ink. They are victims of altered attitudes about themselves and their situation, which cause powerful feelings of hopelessness to abound. Doctors can protect them from these attitudes by providing information, guidance, and support all along the way. Dr. Kevorkian, however, trades upon the vulnerabilities and mental disorders of these patients and in so doing makes a mockery of medicine as a discipline of informed concern for patients.

Let us turn to Dr. Kevorkian, the agent of this epidemic in Michigan, and consider why I think that he is "certifiably" insane, by which I mean that he suffers from a mental condition rendering him dangerous to others.

Without question, Dr. Kevorkian has proved himself dangerous, having participated in killing more than forty people already, with no end in sight. Dr. Kevorkian, by the way, does not shy from the word *killing.* He prescribes it and even coined a term for his practice— *medicide,* that is: "the termination of life performed by . . . professional medical personnel (such as a doctor, nurse, paramedic, physician's assistant, or medical technologist)" (*Prescription: Medicide,* 1991, 202). (Note his sense of a whole industry of killing to come, with much of it to be carried out by technicians because the doctors are busy.)

The question is whether his behavior is a product of a mental disorder. Not everyone agrees on an answer. Indeed, the *British Medical Journal (BMJ)* described Dr. Kevorkian as a "hero."

His champions see no discernible motive for Dr. Kevorkian other than that he believes his work is fitting. The *BMJ* notes that greed for money or fame or some sadistic urge does not motivate Dr. Kevorkian. The editors of the journal make much of the fact that he does not charge a fee for killing. Because of the absence of such motives, they presume that he is a hero among doctors, since it is only a "personal code of honor that admits of no qualification" that leads him into action.

But let us look rather more closely at "personal codes that admit no qualification." We have seen a few of them before, and not all were admirable. As Dr. Kevorkian motors around Michigan carrying cylinders of carbon monoxide or bottles of potassium chloride to dispatch the sick, his is the motivation of a person with an "overvalued idea," a diagnostic formulation first spelled out by the psychiatrist Carl Wernicke in 1906. Wernicke differentiated overvalued ideas from obsessions and delusions. Overvalued ideas are often at the motivational heart of "personal codes that admit no qualification" and certainly provide a drive as powerful as that of hunger for money, fame, or sexual gratification.

An individual with an overvalued idea is someone who has taken up an idea shared by others in his or her milieu or culture and transformed it into a ruling passon or "monomania." It becomes the goal of all this person's efforts, and he or she is prepared to sacrifice everything—family, reputation, health, even life itself—for it. Such people presume that what they do in its service is right regardless of any losses that they or others suffer for it. They see all opposition as at best misguided and at worst malevolent.

For Dr. Kevorkian, people may die before their time, and the fabric of their families may be torn apart, but it's all for the good if he can presume they were "suffering pain unnecessarily" and he has eliminated it. He scorns all opposition—in particular, constitutional democratic opposition—as resting on bad faith or ignorance. Empowered by his idea, he feels free to disregard the law and any of its officers.

An overvalued idea has three characteristics: (1) it is a self-dominating but not idiosyncratic opinion, given great importance by (2) intense emotional feelings over its significance and evoking (3) persistent behavior in its service. For Dr. Kevorkian, thinking about how to terminate the sick has become his exclusive concern. His belief in the justice of his ideas is intense enough for him to starve himself if thwarted by law.

Dr. Kevorkian thinks that all opposition to him is "bad faith" and thus worthy of contempt—a contempt he expresses with no reservation. He is fond of saying that the judicial system of our country is "corrupt," the religious members of our society are "irrational," the medical profession is "insane," the press is "meretricious."

He considers his own behavior "humanitarian." Dr. Kevorkian holds himself beyond reproach, even after killing one patient he believed had multiple sclerosis but whose autopsy revealed no evidence of that disease and another patient with the vague condition "chronic fatigue syndrome" in whom no pathological process could be found at autopsy—only Kevorkian's poison. He acts without taking a careful medical history, trying alternative treatments, or reflecting on how his actions affect such people as surviving family members.

Dr. Kevorkian's is a confident business. As the news reports flow out of Michigan, it appears that his threshold for medicide is getting lower. Physician-assisted suicide that had previously demanded an incurable disease such as Alzheimer's is now practiced upon patients with such chronic complaints as pelvic pain and emphysema, whose life expectancy cannot be specified. He can justify the active termination of anyone with an ailment—which is just what might be expected once the boundary against active killing by doctors has been breached. What's to stop him now that juries have found his actions to be de facto legal in Michigan?

A crucial aspect of overvalued ideas is that, in contrast to delusions, they are not idiosyncratic. They are ideas that can be found in a proportion of the public—often an influential proportion. It is from such reservoirs of opinion that the particular individual harnesses and amplifies an idea with the disproportionate zeal characteristic of a ruling passion. That Dr. Kevorkian can find people in the highest places—even within the medical profession—to support his ideas and say that they see heroism in his actions is not surprising given the passion of the contemporary debate over euthanasia. In this way the person with the overvalued idea may be seen, by those who share his or her opinion but not his or her self-sacrificing zeal, as giving expression to their hopes—disregarding the slower processes of democracy, filled with prejudice against all who resist, and pumped up with a sense of a higher purpose and justice.

People such as Dr. Kevorkian have found a place in history. With some, with the passage of time, we come to agree with the idea, if not the method by which the idea was first expressed. Such was John Brown, the abolitionist, ready to hack five anonymous farmers to death in the Pottawatomie massacre to advance his cause. With others we may come to tolerate some aspect of the idea but see its expression in actual behavior as ludicrous. Such was Carry Nation, the scourge of Kansas barkeeps and boozers, who went to jail hundreds of times for chopping up saloons with a small hatchet in the cause of temperance. With still others, we come to recognize the potential for horror in an overvalued idea held by a person in high authority. Such was Adolf Hitler.

But how is it that anxieties and confusions about medical practice and death can so afflict the judicious people of Michigan as to paralyze them before the outrageous behavior of Dr. Kevorkian and thus generate an environment for this epidemic? In Michigan these states of mind derive from conflicting concerns over medical decisions. The citizens—like any inexpert group—are relatively uninformed about what doctors can do for patients, even in extreme situations. Conflicting goals and unfamiliar practices—common enough around medical decisions—produce anxiety and confusion every time.

No one thinks happily about dying, especially dying in pain. Death is bad; dying can be worse. People who say they do not fear dying—and all the pain and suffering tied to it—have probably not experienced much in life.

This concern, though, certainly has been exaggerated in our times, even though now much can be done to relieve the heaviest burdens of terminally ill patients. Yet through a variety of sources—such as movies, newspapers, and essays—all the negative aspects of dying have been emphasized, the agonies embellished, and the loss of control represented by disease accentuated. Horror stories feed upon one another, and rumors of medical lack of interest grow into opinions that doctors both neglect the dying and hold back relief. Doctors are regularly accused of surrendering to professional taboos or to legal advice to avoid risk of malpractice or prosecution—and in this way are presumed ready to sacrifice their patients out of selfish fear for themselves.

On the contrary, most doctors try to collaborate with patients and do listen to their wishes, especially when treatments that carry painful burdens are contemplated. As Dr. Kevorkian can demonstrate—with videotapes, no less—the patients he killed asked him repeatedly for help in dying rather than for help in living. Do not they have some right to die at their own hand steadied by Dr. Kevorkian? Is not the matter of assisted suicide simply a matter of rights and wants to which any citizen of Michigan is entitled?

The idea of a right to suicide provokes most psychiatrists. Psychiatry has worked to teach everyone that suicide is not an uncomplicated, voluntary act to which rights attach. It has shown that suicide is an act provoked, indeed compelled, by mental disorder—such as a disorienting depression or a set of misdirected, even delusionary, ideas. In that sense psychiatry taught that suicidal people were not "responsible" for this behavior—no matter what they said or wrote in final letters or testaments—any more than they would be for epileptic seizures.

This idea—generated from the careful study of the clinical circumstances and past histories of suicidal patients—gradually prevailed in civil law and even in the canon law of churches. As a result, laws against suicide were repealed—not to make suicide a "right" but to remove it from the status of a crime.

We psychiatrists thought we had done a worthy thing for our society, for families of patients, and even for patients themselves. We were not saying, not for a moment, that we approved of suicide. Far from it. We knew such deaths to be ugly and misguided—misguided in particular because the disposition to die, the wish for suicide, was, on inspection, often a symptom of the very mental disorders that psychiatry treats. Suicide in almost all cases is as far from a rational

choice based on a weighing of the balance books of life as is responding to hallucinated voices or succumbing to the paranoid ideas of a
charismatic madman such as Jim Jones, who at Jonestown directed a
gruesome exhibition of mass assisted suicide.)

Psychiatrists were united in their views about suicide and shook
their heads when contemplating past traditions in which suicides were
considered scandalous. We did not think too deeply about the consequences of our actions. For, after suicide ceased to be a crime, it soon
became a right and, conceivably under some circumstances, such as
when costs of care grow onerous, an obligation. Psychiatrists, who had
worked for decades demonstrating that suicides were insane acts, are
now recruited in Holland to assure that requests for suicide made by
patients offered "no hope of cure" by their doctors are "rational."

What had begun as an effort at explanation and understanding of
the tragic act of suicide has developed into complicity in the seduction of vulnerable people into that very behavior. The patients are
seduced just as the victims in Jonestown were—by isolating them,
sustaining their despair, revoking alternatives, stressing examples of
others choosing to die, and sweetening the deadly poison by speaking
of death with dignity. If even psychiatrists succumb to this complicity
with death, what can be expected of the lay public in Michigan?

At the heart of the confusion lies the contention that if the aim of
medicine is to eliminate suffering and if only the killing of the patient
will relieve the suffering, then killing is justified. On this logic rests
Dr. Kevorkian's repeatedly successful defense before the juries of
Michigan.

Yet the aim of medicine cannot simply be to prevent suffering. Not
only would that be an impossible task, given the nature of human life,
but it would diminish the scope of human potential—almost all of
which demands some travail. The elimination of suffering is a vet-
erinary rather than a medical goal. But veterinarians eliminate their
animal subjects for reasons other than suffering. This fact can occasionally startle us.

When the race horse Cavonnier, second in the 1996 Kentucky
Derby, pulled up lame during the Belmont Stakes later in the year,
everyone watching on television feared that he must have broken a
bone in his leg, with the inevitable consequences. His trainer provided brief comfort when he came on television to describe what had

turned out to be a ligamentous rather than a bony injury to the animal. "This will probably end his racing career" he noted, "but it is not a life-threatening injury." He then paused before adding, "However, he *is* a gelding." An ominous comment for Cavonnier and one worth remembering when anyone says, in defense of killing infirm people, "They shoot horses, don't they?" They do, but for many reasons other than just to protect horses from suffering. Sometimes it's to save money. Are we ready for the Cavonnier test for ourselves?

The idea that diseases herald only mortality and death, to be hurried along if their burdens are overwhelming, is not only an ethical error but a fundamental misunderstanding of contemporary medical science. Contemporary physician-scientists do not think of diseases as "entities," "things," "maledictions," and, in this sense, signposts to the grave but as processes in life for which the body has ways of compensating and resisting, even if only temporarily. Diseases, in this way, are construed as forms of life under altered circumstances rather than as modes of death.

Because diseases are processes rather than entities, efforts to sustain life, alleviate symptoms, and moderate impairments represent collaborations with nature itself. These efforts remain the essence of doctoring, the whole reason for investing in the study of diseases and the body's responses to them. Physician-assisted suicide and euthanasia attack the very premises on which medical science and practice are progressing today and do so by denying the life that scientific conceptions of disease represent. Life with dignity—not death with dignity—is what doctors aim for in their practice and in their science.

Medicine is one of the practical arts—a fact old enough to be known to Aristotle—among which are included navigation, economics, and architecture and for which the goal is usually obvious and unquestioned. For medicine, actions to prevent, alleviate, and cure are aimed at the obvious goal of sustaining the life and health of patients. Technical progress through scientific discoveries assists these actions, rendering them more effective. But modern techniques can seem in some circumstances to forestall the inevitable, prolong suffering, deny reality with little or no gain to the patient. Dr. Kevorkian writes and disseminates stories on this theme to justify his actions and to bolster his support. Allow me to present a story in which the conflict between preserving life and surrendering to disease was resolved by doctors who recognized their limits while striving to facilitate and extend a person's best experiences.

Nelson Butters was one of America's most distinguished neuropsychologists of the past twenty-five years. He died in 1995 at age fifty-eight after suffering for just under three years from the nightmare known as Lou Gehrig disease. This disease is a relentless and progressive wasting of the body because of an atrophic degeneration of the nerves that innervate the muscles. As the body wastes away over the course of months, the mind is customarily unaffected and witnesses these depredations. It anticipates further weakness and ultimate death from a loss of strength to breathe. Such an affliction you would not wish on your worst enemy. Dr. Jack Kevorkian lives to terminate—the earlier the better—any patient smitten by it.

My colleague and friend Nelson Butters saw it through to its natural end. In so doing—without making it his mission—he rebuked those who cannot (or will not) differentiate incurable diseases, of which there are many, from untreatable patients, of which there are few.

Nelson was a great scientist and an indomitable man. He took on all of life's challenges, personal and professional, with vigor and courage. But when he learned that he had Lou Gehrig disease, he was shaken and responded with a most natural discouragement. "I'd rather die than be helpless," he said several times to his doctors. Yet he proved willing to try the assistance they offered him at each of the bad patches in his course, so that he could continue to enjoy what remained despite his illness. He had neurologists aiding him with his growing weakness, and he had psychiatrists and psychologists ready to assist him when he was tormented by his prospects.

He had bad times. They came mostly when some partial surrender to the disease was required—accepting a wheelchair, retreating to bed, undergoing a tracheostomy to facilitate breathing—but after each procedure, and despite its implicit indication that his condition was progressing, he recovered his cheer as he found himself more comfortable and able to continue his work with students and colleagues and his life with his family.

Like Stephen Hawking, Nelson toward the end made use of computers to communicate and work. This permitted him to edit a major journal in neuropsychology, even when he could move only one finger and then only one toe. With these small movements he used e-mail to write to colleagues everywhere—usually on professional matters but also to transmit amusing academic gossip.

Eventually, Nelson lost all his strength. He was left with only eye-blinking signals, breathing with the help of a machine. Then he asked his doctors, with his family around him, that the ventilator cease breathing for him. This was done, and on a weekend he slipped into a coma and died—thirty-four months after his symptoms began.

Nelson, his family, and his doctors had achieved much together. They fought to enable him to sustain purposeful life as long as possible. They weathered distressing, powerfully painful portions of his clinical course. The doctors never suggested a poison to shorten his life. When there was still something to do, they encouraged him to try to do it and helped allay his reluctance at the prospect. And in the end they surrendered to the illness without betraying their mission or letting contemporary technology drag them along.

It was grim. Everyone who knew him was saddened to think that Nelson had to suffer so. But everyone also was struck by how he overcame the disease by staying purposeful, lively, and wittily intelligent right through to the end, teaching much to all of us.

I tell this story because many believe that permitting a progressive infirmity to continue right out to its natural end is cruel and pointless. It certainly is tough. Any gains need to be identified. In fact, the gains for Nelson Butters were several.

Most obvious among them was the continuation of Nelson's work as a scientist, an editor, and a teacher for many months, despite his illness. This was no trivial gain, for he was an inventive scientist with deep insight into his discipline. He continued to function effectively and to enjoy his work and the accomplishments of his students.

Another gain was an extended duration of Nelson's company to his family and his friends. Again, no trivial matter, for he was a lovable person. One of his daughters decided to help nurse him through his trials, and after his death, reflecting on all she had seen and done, she decided to take up a career in nursing incapacitated people.

Finally, there was the appreciation—to the point of amazement—on the part of his doctors of the value he fashioned from their efforts to help him. They told me how he had taken what they offered and made more of it—more than they expected and more in the form of continuing work and personal life—than they thought could be achieved. This was as true of the neurologists who offered means to offset his physical impairments as it was of the psychiatrists who at times of particular discouragement helped him keep going.

These gains were made easier because Nelson was such a good man and had such a good family to support him. Yet I sensed the awe felt by the doctors themselves for what had been accomplished in the end. Almost despite themselves and their own feelings about this awful disease, they had been partners with Nelson in a great achievement. They had carried out excellently the task set before doctors— help the patient encounter and resist the chaos of disease for as long as possible—and thus preserve the purposeful character of life to its end.

In Nelson's life a set of interwoven but distinct purposes—husband, father, teacher, scientist—were sustained by him with the help of several doctors. And this happened despite the depredations of a crushing disease and the recurrent waves of discouragement that naturally accompany the loss of vitality and the realization of impending death.

But there was something more in Nelson's story. For all that he was surrounded by devoted nurses, technicians, family, and physicians, death came to him alone just as it will to each of us. Its approach confronts us all with the challenge to decide what moves us, what matters most, what we love. Nelson loved life. He wanted as much of it as he could have. Through this love he won a victory over death— for himself, for his family, for all who knew him.

This is really what distinguishes him from Dr. Kevorkian, his sad victims, and those who support his cause. None of them love life the way Nelson did—not enough, certainly, to work hard and suffer much for it, not enough to appreciate it throughout its course, when it flickers just as much as when it glows. And certainly not enough to realize that sometimes we need help to protect it so that we don't throw it away.

To be on the side of life provides a source of sanity. Be on the side of life and your course is clear, your efforts concentrated, the rules coherent. Bad patches can then be overcome, and even bad luck such as befell my friend Nelson Butters can be turned into something good. Be on the side of death and things fall apart, chaos reigns, and the fearful passions evoked by conflicting aims make malice, misdirection, sentiment, and compassion all look the same.

One can think of ways to combat the deadly convergence of madnesses in Michigan and to deter the spread of this local epidemic to other regions of our country. The suicidal patients certainly should be treated for their depressive vulnerabilities by doctors able to assist them with their underlying illnesses. Dr. Kevorkian, the agent of their extinction, should be stopped by whatever means the state has at its disposal to stay dangerous men. And the people of Michigan should be taught about the capacities of modern medicine. With this information, the hope is, they will emerge from their anxious confusions, accept mortality for what it is rather than for what they imagine, and, at last, end their support for this insanity.

The American Scholar, 1997

Dying Made Easy

Two factors determine how people die: the diseases they have, and who they are. In any given case, these two factors vary in salience. With sudden, terminal diseases like massive heart attacks or apoplectic cerebral hemorrhages, the disease dominates, and mostly obliterates, personality. Then does the power of nature, the "great equalizer," render alike the death of rich and poor, wise and foolish, brave and timid.

But with slowly advancing disorders—cancer, liver failure, AIDS—who you are powerfully affects how you die. Temperament and character, apprehensions and commitments, resources and support, shape the response to symptoms. Indeed, from the point of view of society, the behavior of one patient suffering from an incurable disease can differ so radically from that of another suffering from the same disease as to influence our attitudes toward life and death themselves.

In medicine, these are commonplace ideas; the individuality of patients with similar diseases was emphasized as long ago as Hippocrates. But they have achieved a new resonance with the recent debates over euthanasia and assisted suicide and with widespread popular concern over easing the final stages of life for the terminally ill.

Two cases in particular commend themselves to our attention. The first is that of Thomas Youk of Michigan, who in the fall of 1998 was killed by Dr. Jack Kevorkian. This act of euthanasia was recorded on videotape and, on Sunday, November 22, witnessed by more than sixteen million people on the CBS news program *60 Minutes*. The second case is that of Morris S. Schwartz, a former professor of sociology at Brandeis University and the eponymous subject of *Tuesdays with Morrie* (1997) by Mitch Albom, a book that has been on the *New York Times* best-seller list, mostly in the number-one position, for more than a year.

What connects the two cases is that both men were suffering from the same neurological disease: amyotrophic lateral sclerosis (ALS), commonly referred to as Lou Gehrig disease after the great New York

Yankee first baseman who died from it. And yet, though they had identical afflictions, the contrast in the final moments of their lives could not have been sharper. The first man's death was ghastly: Kevorkian prepared the site by persuading the patient's family to leave home for a few hours, and then, when he had him alone, he killed him by intravenous injection of a poison to stop his heart. By contrast, Morris Schwartz, whose advance through the terminal stages of ALS is almost as well recorded as that of Thomas Youk, died naturally and in peace, surrounded by friends and family.

Each of these two deaths thus makes a cultural statement. Judging those statements, however, is not quite so straightforward an exercise as it might appear.

Other than how he died, we know very little about Thomas Youk. He was a Catholic; he restored and raced vintage cars; he was said to have led an active life. Members of his family, who spoke about him on *60 Minutes*, described him as a "fighter."

Youk had been suffering from ALS for two years. His family called Kevorkian because, they reported, he was "in terrible pain, had trouble breathing and swallowing, and was choking on his own saliva." On his first visit, Kevorkian performed the most cursory of medical examinations, confirming only that Youk showed severe paralysis of the limbs and had difficulty breathing and speaking. Concluding that he was "terrified of choking," Kevorkian had him sign a consent form for euthanasia, "to be administered by a competent medical professional in order to end with certainty my intolerable and hopelessly incurable suffering." Two nights later, he returned to do the job.

It was, of course, not his first killing. Over the past decade, Kevorkian has been actively soliciting people to enable him to "assist" them in committing suicide, going so far as to advertise his services in newspapers. By means of a device—his so-called Mercitron—capable of delivering intravenous poison when the patient presses an activating button, he has fostered the deaths of more than 130 people. He defends his behavior as "symptom" relief—his treatments, he says, are not intended to kill but to relieve the patient's distress—although his favorite medication, potassium chloride, has no role in the relief of symptoms other than by stopping the heart. This justification has nevertheless satisfied three juries before whom he has been tried for murder.

When asked by a Michigan paper if Youk had had any last words, Kevorkian, the physician closest to him in his final days, replied, "I don't know. I never understood a thing he said." What he did know was that Youk and his family had reached their self-proclaimed limits in tolerating the symptoms of disease. And that, for his purposes, was enough. For what Kevorkian was seeking and had found in Youk was an individual who could be used to challenge the laws of Michigan against euthanasia as he had previously challenged the state law against assisted suicide. His true intent, in other words, had less to do with relieving the suffering of an individual than with making euthanasia, as he has put it, a "fundamental American right—part of life, liberty and the pursuit of happiness." Youk was a means to that end.

If we know little about the man who agreed to become Kevorkian's "poster boy for euthanasia," as Mike Wallace referred to Thomas Youk on *60 Minutes*, we know a very great deal about Morris Schwartz. Not only was he a well-regarded sociologist with many publications to his name, but his dying and death were the subject of more than this one book, *Tuesdays with Morrie*. ABC-TV's news program *Nightline* had interviewed him three times over the two-year course of his illness, and television viewers had come to appreciate his lively and brave demeanor. It was, indeed, the first of these broadcasts on *Nightline* that impelled Mitch Albom, a sportswriter for the *Detroit Free Press* who had studied with Schwartz at Brandeis, to begin visiting his former teacher weekly at his home outside Boston. Not only did Albom go on to write a best-seller about that experience, but Schwartz's aphorisms on sickness and death have also been collected in another book, *Letting Go: Morrie's Reflections on Living While Dying* (1996).

Tuesdays with Morrie is a small book—192 pages long. It begins by describing Morrie's life before his illness and the circumstances in which he and Mitch met. (Everyone goes by a nickname or a diminutive in this book—not only "Morrie" and "Mitch" but "Rob," "Gordie," "Charlie," even "Rabbi Al.") Then, in a series of fourteen chapters, we are given vignettes of the Tuesday visits. Through this record of the conversations between the two men, we become progressively enlightened as to Morrie's attitudes toward dying and death as well as toward such matters as the expenditure of emotion, forgiveness, family, and regret. The final chapter describes Morrie's death and funeral.

Although *Tuesdays with Morrie* is mainly a vehicle for Morrie to speak about his illness and himself, we also learn about Mitch and his family and about Mitch's reactions to the progress of his friend's disease. The events of the sickroom and the way he and Morrie cope with them are graphically rendered, as are the suffering and death of an uncle of Mitch's from pancreatic cancer. (Mitch's younger brother, to whom the book is dedicated, has the same disease.) The net effect is to give us a picture of life in the round and to bring home the blessed appropriateness of being able to die as we have lived— surrounded by friends, exchanging affectionate thoughts.

I will return in a moment to what, in Morrie's case, those thoughts are. But it may be useful first to say something about the illness to which Morris Schwartz and Thomas Youk responded in so divergent a manner.

ALS is a grim, incurable, progressive neurological disease characterized by a gradual degeneration of the nerves that activate the muscles of the body. Its first symptoms can appear anywhere—in the arms or legs or around the mouth and jaw. But eventually and gradually it afflicts the entire body with a total atrophy of the muscles, ending in complete paralysis. Death comes from the weakening of the respiratory action of the chest and diaphragm, making breathing ineffective; if the patient is not maintained on a respirator, he or she will slip into a coma and die.

Although ALS is an illness that no one would wish on another, it is not the worst illness from which to die. Unlike, say, pancreatic cancer (of the kind Mitch describes his uncle and brother as suffering from), ALS is relatively painless. It does produce much discomfort from coughing and from the aching of limbs that cannot change their position, but these can be ameliorated by good nursing care. The end itself is quiet. The muscles of respiration fail very slowly, and the patient usually has no sense of smothering but rather is gradually narcotized from the accumulation of carbon dioxide. Death often comes at night; the patient may fall asleep in the evening with no obvious change in his or her condition and then just fail to awaken.

Moreover, in contrast to other incurable diseases, ALS does not produce delusional depressions of the kind that can crush the spirit by triggering attitudes of self-blame, hopelessness, and a profound sense of the meaninglessness of all human action. These depressions, which derive from the brain disorders that can accompany AIDS and Huntington or Parkinson disease, are unresponsive to efforts at distraction. They represent a form of insanity that can provoke suicide and that demands psychopharmacologic attention.

This is hardly to say that patients with ALS are not often discouraged or greatly dismayed. Such symptoms are reported frequently in *Tuesdays with Morrie*, and the family of Thomas Youk also suggested that he was suffering from them. But moods of this nature differ in kind from delusional depression and are more properly thought of as aspects of demoralization: emotional reactions, provoked by actual circumstances, that everyone has experienced in minor or major forms in life and that can be relieved by thoughtful psychological assistance, professional and amateur alike. Many patients with ALS can throw off their sad feelings for long periods of time, just as Morrie did—sometimes through their own efforts, usually with help from others who understand them and what they are undergoing.

Another vital characteristic of ALS is that its victims have no loss of cognitive power. Nothing in the disease prevents them from thinking and planning as before. Conceivably, this in itself can become a burden, since patients are alert to the relentless progress of their disease toward death. But in many cases, the retention of cognitive power offers a means of helping them. Morrie, for example, was promptly informed of his future when the diagnosis of ALS was made; although his intense awareness of his fate did bring on intermittent feelings of demoralization, his clarity of mind permitted him to take charge of his situation, put aside self-pity, and undertake activities that encouraged him and gave him purpose.

Patients with ALS can do valuable work. Mayor Fiorello La Guardia made Lou Gehrig an officer of the New York City Parole Board after the Yankees—true to type, even then—cut him off once he could no longer play. He worked effectively at that job for a year. Steven Hawking, the famous professor of astronomy at Cambridge University who suffers from a more slowly progressive form of ALS, continues to do cosmological research, write, and teach with the help of advanced electronic devices. Nelson Butters, one of the most talented and productive American neuropsychologists of recent decades, edited journals and supervised psychological research right up until the last weeks of his life.

An especially ironic example is offered by the case of Noel David Earley of Rhode Island, who in 1996 began to demand euthanasia for his advancing condition and found a health worker to provide a syringe with which he might commit suicide. The date on which Earley planned to kill himself, he announced, was December 4, 1996—a date still far enough in the future as to give him ample time to tell his story and protest the laws forbidding euthanasia. In the intervening months he testified before the state government and the Rhode Island Medical Society and contacted the American Civil Liberties Union to gain its help in asserting his "right to die"; he was given plenty of airtime and plenty of ink. But when December 4 finally came, Earley decided he had not adequately explained his position. He thereupon set a new date several weeks ahead. Friends now had to carry his shrunken and paralyzed body around his apartment and to interviews at which he continued his protest against the state of Rhode Island and its uncivilized laws.

Finally, after a second postponement of his announced self-murder, Earley unexpectedly died in his sleep. Friends said he would surely have killed himself eventually, and they themselves were surely prepared to fight for his "right" to do so. But many also conceded that he had been at his most cheerful when crusading against the laws that deprived him of this right; he was never so chipper as when fighting to die.

The lesson is simple. ALS is a bleak condition, but give a person who has it a reason to live, and he or she will keep going to the end, distressed intermittently by its burdens but aided by any sense of purpose and grateful for any help. And that, indeed, is where medicine enters the picture. Specialist physicians know the progress and succession of symptoms and the treatments that can relieve them. Skilled nurses can administer daily care—delivery of medications, bathing and cleaning the body, managing the environment of the home or hospital room—in ways that mitigate both the symptoms of the disease and its psychological complications.

No such attendance followed poor Thomas Youk. Jack Kevorkian, it is important to note, was trained as a pathologist and had no practical experience in caring for terminally ill patients before he embarked on his crusade to become their deliverer. He takes his moral authority, moreover, not from his role as a doctor but, as I have already suggested, from political ideology—and specifically from his understanding of the libertarian philosophies of John Stuart Mill, Thomas Jefferson, and John Locke. What more fundamental right, he asks, than the right to decide when to die? If, under the constraints of disease and suffering, "you don't have liberty and self-determination," he proclaimed on *60 Minutes*, "you got nothing."

All this, however, is a lie built on a terrible distortion. The distortion has to do with the way Kevorkian drags his ideological heroes—Locke, Jefferson, Mill, and the rest—into a realm in which their political categories do not apply. As hard as it may be to tell the difference between "true" and "alienated" desires when we are in full possession of our physical and mental faculties, it is a thousand times harder when outside forces overwhelm the self, rendering it vulnerable to unreflective impulses. Among the reasons patients with dire illnesses turn to physicians for help is that their capacities for thinking and planning have been compromised. The responsibility for drawing distinctions under these circumstances lies at the very heart of medical practice. It is the duty doctors owe their patients.

In any case—and here is the lie—the real philosophy espoused by Kevorkian is a doctrine not of *rights* but of *feelings*. For in dismissing the role of the physician as a provider of reasoned guidance, as one who helps a patient differentiate good from bad, right from wrong, responsible decisions from impulses, Kevorkian "privileges" instead the momentary inclinations of the patient, who is most often in extremis. Kevorkian himself never reviews a patient's full history; never considers the relief of symptoms, other than via death; never invokes contemporary medical knowledge concerning the management of a patient's disease; and never reflects on the patient's mental state or personal vulnerabilities. He also never considers how his own proposals and practices may influence a suggestible patient's decisions. The propositions advanced by unsettled and possibly unbalanced minds he absurdly equates with the thoughts of free and reflective citizens, and upon these unbalanced minds he then grandly confers their "rights."

What we are talking about, then, is a special kind of nihilism and a special kind of atomism. In the Kevorkian worldview, the patient is a solitary figure, related to nothing or no one beyond him- or herself, with neither a past to honor nor a future to influence (a future, that is, distinct from his impending death). The patient's desires, regardless of their sources and implications, regardless of how they might be affected by cool reflection or alleviating therapy, are the only factors that count. A man named Thomas Youk complains that he is tired of life under the conditions he faces; his family agrees; without studying the circumstances out of which these feelings were generated, and against which they might be evaluated, a man named Dr. Kevorkian kills him.

How have we, as a culture, come to this pass? In a narrow sense, the question is easily answered. When we—doctors, family, and friends— endorse a patient's feelings of discouragement, treating them as the most pertinent fact about him and leaving him without suggestions or plans for acting purposefully during what remains of his life, then we open the door to Kevorkianism. But surely—the reader may protest—we do not all act so callously. Thank goodness, no one ever thought of abusing Morrie Schwartz the way Thomas Youk was abused; and that makes all the difference in the world. The culture may not yet be so lost.

But we cannot really leave it at that. For the fact is that, in its own determinedly upbeat way, *Tuesdays with Morrie* is a disheartening book. True, for people seeking commonsense instruction, it may serve—from its sales figures, it clearly does serve—a useful purpose, akin to the purpose served, for the beginnings of life, by Dr. Benjamin Spock's famous book on baby and child care. Between them, Morrie and Mitch also offer lots of good advice of a more general nature. They tell us to accept with grace the loss of dignity that accompanies serious illness: the odors and minor ugliness of the sickroom. They tell us to take our friendships seriously and to make efforts and sacrifices to preserve them. And the like.

But their limitations are evident and in the end disqualifying. Like Dr. Spock, Morrie and Mitch are strong on the hows and debilitatingly weak on the whys. As a professor, Morrie comes from the "group-process" school of social psychology—a doctrine that promotes a kind of therapy based on the vigorous exchange of off-the-cuff personal interpretations and frank, uncensored opinions. He seems (again like Dr. Spock) most at home in the 1960s, a time when talk and self-display took on a life of their own and universities were transformed overnight from places where one learned what was known into places where the point was to *discuss* everything.

Discussion, indeed, is the keynote of *Tuesdays with Morrie*, if *discussion* is not too elevated a word for the psychobabble, mixed in equal parts of crude Marxism and empty hedonism, that fills its pages. Throughout, Morrie and Mitch talk about the defects of "our culture" (their term), deprecating it like a couple of old hippies. "We work too hard and are too ambitious," opines Morrie one Tuesday. Or, "Money is a substitute for love for most people." Or, "As I'm sitting here dying neither money nor power will give you the feeling you're looking for." Asked what might give you that feeling, he replies: "Devote yourself to creating something that gives you purpose and meaning." Such as? Morrie does not say, and Mitch never thinks to ask.

"Accept what you are able to do and what you are not able to do." "Learn to forgive yourself and others." Never "assume it's too late to get involved." How the agonizing choices life puts before us can be negotiated, and tragic errors avoided, on the basis of such empty maxims is never examined by Morrie or Mitch. Their vocabulary is heavy on words like *love, openness, compromise, "feelings"*; light on *duty, responsibility, accountability.*▲ What one especially misses in *Tuesdays with Morrie*, a book devoted to the subject of death, is any sense of awe in its presence.

The mystery of human existence—so poignantly felt by everyone at the great moments of birth, marriage, and death—is passed over by our two protagonists without so much as a murmur. At one point, Mitch asks Morrie his opinion of the biblical figure of Job and of the God Who "made him suffer." Morrie responds: "I think, God overdid it." From a dying man who is himself showing considerable Job-like perseverance, this is a witty remark. Unfortunately, when it comes to interpreting life and death, neither here nor elsewhere does this highly educated man stop to ponder the great questions posed by Job,

▲In writing this book about Lou Gehrig disease, Mitch Albom, who has been voted America's number-one sports columnist ten times by his colleagues, tellingly misquotes Gehrig's farewell speech at Yankee Stadium on July 4, 1939. Gehrig said: "Today I consider myself the luckiest man on the face of the earth." Albom has him saying: "Today I *feel* like the luckiest man on the face of the earth" (emphasis added). This little slip is of the essence of the solipsism that infects *Tuesdays with Morrie*.

not least among them the question of whether there is anything beyond ourselves that can judge us and our purposes or imbue the choices we make with permanent significance.

"Naked I came from my mother's womb, naked I shall return. The Lord gave, the Lord has taken away. Blessed be the name of the Lord." Between Job's dispassionate but sublimely *connected* thought and Morrie's anodyne one-liners stretches an unbridgeable spiritual chasm.

Does it matter? Morrie, after all, died the way he lived. He was jovial and spirited; he hung in there; he lives on in the minds of his friends. So what if he talked a fair amount of nonsense along the way?

The real question, though, is whether any lasting strength can be gained from an account like this one—strength that derives from knowing ourselves (as Morrie and Mitch do not) to be the legatees of inviolable traditions, cultural and professional alike, as well as members of a vast and enduring human community that stretches back into history and forward into the experience of those yet to come. Morrie's method of managing his own death is not to be disparaged. It worked for him, thanks to his innate pluck and to the special arrangements available for his care. But how is that method, untied to principle, to tradition, or to any sense of larger human obligation, going to help those who lack his advantages: the weak as well as the strong, the lonely as well as the befriended, the tortured as well as the pain-free?

To the proponents of euthanasia and assisted suicide, the attitudes expressed in *Tuesdays with Morrie* offer, alas, no prescriptive resistance. They can be no more than a sweet interlude, a brief way station along the path paved by Dr. Kevorkian—and by all the kinder and gentler Kevorkians who are waiting a step or two behind. On that path, the signpost, brief and desolating, reads: You are alone.

Commentary, 1999

Annihilating Terri Schiavo

During the tumultuous final weeks in the life of Terri Schiavo, the young woman who died in a Florida hospice in April, press reports in the nation's media typically focused on the bitter conflicts among members of her family over her treatment, disagreements among consultants over her state of consciousness, and the increasingly intense arguments in legislatures and the courts over her guardianship. Since her death, the case and the story of her death and dying have been mined for their bearing on our ongoing culture wars and for the debate over the place of "values" in our politics. In particular, the seeming failure of the Republican leadership to rally legislative support in favor of keeping her alive has been seized upon as evidence of the Right's overreaching and as a lesson in the ironies of ideology. In the words of a writer in the April 24, 2005, *New York Times Magazine,* "the heirs to Goldwater and Reagan seemed to forget how they came to control the values debate in America in the first place: not by interfering in the moral choices of families but by promising to *stop* government from doing exactly that."

Many a hidden assumption lurks in that statement, not least concerning the (assumed) wishes of the dying woman herself. It is worth reminding ourselves, moreover, that she succumbed in the end by being deprived of food and water by order of the courts—which is to say, by order of government. But in what follows I want to concentrate on another, neglected aspect of this entire dismal episode.

Conspicuously missing from the chorus of voices arguing over the meaning and implications of the Schiavo case have been the views of a class of people with a uniquely relevant body of experience and insight: namely, the doctors and nurses who customarily provide care to patients like Terri Schiavo. As a result, few people appear to have grasped that the way she died was most unusual. That, instead, it has been widely understood to be not only a proper but also a perfectly commonsensical way to die, a way approved of by most doctors and nurses, can only be explained by a deep change that has taken place over the past decades in our thinking about how to care for the helpless and the disabled among us.

Let us begin with the published facts. In 1990, when Terri Schiavo was in her mid-twenties, she suffered a cardiac arrest that produced a severe cerebral anoxic injury—anoxia being an abnormally low amount of oxygen in the body's tissues—and coma. From this coma she emerged gradually, settling for the next fifteen years into an impaired state of consciousness. She could swallow, breathe, sleep, and awaken without assistance and could react to sudden sounds with a glance or to pain by grimacing or groaning. But she was apathetic to inner needs and external events. She was mute, mostly immobile, incontinent, psychologically blank.

For the past several years, Terri Schiavo was being treated in a hospice for terminally ill people. There she received basic nursing care for her bodily needs—she was bathed and turned on schedule—while nutritious fluids were supplied through a tube that had been inserted through her abdomen into her stomach during her earlier treatment for injury. Because of her immobility and apathy, she gradually developed muscle contractions that twisted her limbs and body into a fixed contorted posture. She suffered frequent bedsores, and, with poor oral hygiene, her teeth rotted. In this state she was sustained by the regular attention of a devoted staff and family, being financially supported by money her husband, Michael, had gained for her through a malpractice suit.

And so she would have remained—alive and physically stable, giving off a few signals that were possibly reflexive but were believed by some members of the hospice staff and her family to represent modest signs of awareness of her surroundings—until, within a period of years, an infection, a blood clot, or a cardio-respiratory difficulty would bring her life to an end. What changed in this situation was not her physical condition but her husband's mind.

He, her legal guardian, had at first battled for her care and support but had gradually lost hope of her further recovery. He first signaled his new attitude when he balked at permitting antibiotic treatment for a recurring bladder infection. Although dissuaded on that occasion by the nursing staff, he eventually began to demand that they stop all sustaining treatments, including the gastric tube that provided nutritious fluids or any feeding of his wife by spoon or cup.

The other parties, however, were not won over to Michael Schiavo's view that Terri was beyond hope of recovery. Instead, her parents launched what became a long legal fight with him for her guardianship. Their own intention was to continue her care in the hospice. At the very least, they wanted to feed her by mouth as one would any helpless person.

Through a series of court battles, legislative enactments, and executive mandates, the husband's right of guardianship was upheld, the gastric tube was removed, and all—hospice staff, parents, siblings, onlookers—were forbidden by court order to give her food or drink orally. Even a chip of ice to relieve the pain of a parched mouth and throat was judicially prohibited, and local sheriffs were alerted to prevent it. Within thirteen distress-filled days, she died of dehydration.

What other factors are relevant here—laboratory data, clinical diagnostic opinions, expressed views to the extent we have been informed of them?

Terri Schiavo's initial cardiac arrest, so rare in a young person, had been provoked by a morbidly low level of potassium in her blood—an unusual metabolic event unless the person has been losing potassium through persistent vomiting, diarrhea, or diuresis (increased discharge of urine). The plausible diagnostic explanation was that she was suffering from bulimia nervosa and had been voluntarily and regularly vomiting to control her body weight.

The injury to her brain was demonstrably extensive. The electroencephalogram (EEG) was grossly abnormal and typical of a patient with severely impaired consciousness. In 2002, a computer-activated tomogram (CAT scan) of her brain showed extensive cavities of dead tissue in both cerebral hemispheres and spotty islands of loss in the band of cerebral cortex remaining around the cavities. But no functional assessments of her surviving cerebral tissue was performed by means of magnetic-resonance imaging (MRI) or positron-emission tomography (PET). The absence of such assessments is surprising. Especially if done serially, they would have demonstrated whether any neural activity persisted in the band of cortex around the cavities and whether any of this tissue was recovering over time.

Terri Schiavo was examined by qualified neurologists. Most of them concluded that she fit into the rather amorphous group of severely brain-injured patients defined as being in a "persistent vegetative state" (PVS). This diagnostic category encompasses individuals with cerebral diseases of various kinds who, though only dimly wakeful, retain the life-sustaining functions of respiration, blood circulation, and metabolic integrity.

It is perhaps because such patients display so lowered a state of vigilance that, in striving to define their condition, neurologists lighted upon a metaphor contrasting vegetation with animation. I remember teasing the admirable clinician who first coined this term that I had seen many patients but few carrots sleeping, waking, grunting, or flinching from pain. Although the term *vegetative* does distinguish what is lost from what remains in such a patient's capacities, it can also have the unfortunate effect of suggesting that there is something less worthy about those in this condition.

As for the adjective *persistent*, it is perfectly precise and makes no prognostic claim (as would, say, the term *permanent*). It simply describes the patient's history. What we know from experience is that, as with most neurological impairments, patients "persisting" in this state of blunted consciousness for more than eighteen months are generally unlikely to recover.

The neurologists who coined the diagnostic category PVS did so out of the best of clinical motives. In particular, they wanted to distinguish it from the "brain-dead" state, where no functional capacities—to breathe, to swallow, or to respond—remain. With "brain death," a patient evinces no response to any stimulus. Brain monitors show no activity. Heart and viscera can carry on their automatic activity only with the aid of mechanical, ventilator-driven respiration and will cease when it is discontinued.

By definition, then, PVS is not death hidden by machinery. It is human life under altered neurological circumstances. And this distinction makes all the difference in how doctors and nurses think about it and treat its sufferers.

The phrase "life under altered circumstances" encompasses every human sickness and disability. It also speaks to what is entailed in the professional art of medicine—the art, that is, of identifying, differentiating, curing, rehabilitating, defending, and, in the words of the Hippocratic oath, "benefit[ing]" the sick. Given that doctors and nurses naturally align themselves with life and are trained to care for whatever life brings, including "life under altered neurological circumstances," it is only to be expected that they would reject and shrink from actions that aim to kill. Exactly how they come to that civilizing point of view in their training to become doctors and nurses is a story unto itself.

The education of doctors and nurses is an interweaving of related but essentially distinct pathways of experience. One pathway comprises accumulated scientific and technical knowledge of the laws of nature. The other pathway is made up of extended, one-on-one experience with patients. This begins early as, with guidance from the masters of their craft, students and interns encounter clinical cases in the form of intensely personal dramas, events shared with many concerned parties: patients, relatives, fellow professionals. In these encounters, all the powers of science and technology that identify the characteristics of "life under altered circumstances" are enriched and elucidated.

As it happens, I have had many years of experience as both student and teacher in caring for patients like Terri Schiavo with neuropsychiatric disorders. My patients have included individuals with dementia, confusion, apathy, and stupor, produced by diseases like Alzheimer's, Huntington's, stroke, infection, trauma, malnutrition, poisoning, and asphyxia. As is true of most doctors, the clinical cases I remember most vividly—right down to the location within a hospital of the bed where the patient lay—were those I saw early in my training.

Such cases help form the assumptions and attitudes that we doctors and nurses bring toward the responsibilities that we have elected to take on. We can always be persuaded to talk about these war stories, as we call them, because they were so important to us in learning our craft and in how we act thereafter toward the people in our care. Here is one such story.

In the late 1950s, I was the resident neurologist on a team responsible for the care of some twenty-five chronically ill, permanently disabled, and bed-bound patients suffering from advanced neuropsychiatric disorders. Each morning I would travel from bed to bed in the company of several junior interns, pushing a cart with the patients' records and checking up on them while simultaneously discoursing on what I knew about their condition. Because patients in

such a chronic setting change little from day to day, finding something new to say about them becomes a challenge.

This was especially true of one patient—a man in his late fifties
who, after a botched brain operation, had been left in an apathetic
state not too different from Terri Schiavo's. Like her, he gave little
evidence of awareness, responding mostly with groans and grimaces
and moving little, if at all. He had been in that state for several years
when I took over on the ward; ultimately, he would live thirteen years
in this condition.

The nurses, who were feeding him with spoon and cup, thought
he had some awareness—as did some relatives who visited him—and
even claimed to have heard him utter a few words. But evidently
their testimony was not taken seriously. A biographical sketch written
about him after his death—for in his active career he had been very
well known—would state that, once having suffered his brain injury,
"he never spoke again."

We young physicians felt honored to be caring for this man, who
was of our fraternity. Prior to his injury, indeed, he had been quite
simply the foremost clinical scientist in America. Among his many
achievements, he had illuminated the functions of the parathyroid
glands and so enlarged scientific knowledge of calcium metabolism,
the dynamics of bone construction, and diseases of the bone like
osteoporosis and osteomalacia. From his specific studies, he had discerned general principles (including "end-organ resistance to hormonal action," a concept prefiguring the receptor revolution in
endocrinology), and he made leaders of his students by teaching
them how to employ biological science in investigating the pathogenesis of human diseases. In a relatively brief academic career, he
had changed the face of American academic medicine and pointed
the way to the future.

So we were pleased to care for him. But this did not ease the task
before me upon visiting his bedside each morning as I searched for
something interesting to say to my jaded interns. Soon enough they
began to grumble that I was repeating myself as I would note duti-
fully that, although Dr. A's apathetic state was profound and un-
changing, occasionally such a patient might, if startled, give out a
coherent response revealing some human consciousness. Looking at
the man lying before them, they thought they had ample reason to

doubt the applicability of my ideas to this case. A particularly bold intern challenged me one morning: "Enough of that, show us that he can respond."

I knew perfectly well that I was being baited over a matter where I was unsure of my ground, but I moved briskly from the records cart to the bed, shook the patient by the shoulder, and asked in a sharp voice: "Dr. A, what's the serum calcium in pseudopseudohypoparathyroidism?" For the first time in my experience with him, he glanced up at me and, loudly enough for all the interns to hear, said: "It's just about normal."

A full and complete sentence had emerged from a man whom none of us had ever heard speak before. His answer was correct—as he should know, having discovered and named the condition I asked him about. Subsequently, in all the months we cared for him, he would never utter another word. But what a difference that moment had made to all of us. We matured that day not only in matters of the mind but in matters of the heart. Somehow, deep inside that body and damaged brain, he was there—and our job was to help him. If we had ever had misgivings before, we would never again doubt the value of caring for people like him. And we didn't give a fig that his EEG was grossly abnormal.

To apply these observations to Terri Schiavo's case, we might imagine her as the subject of a medical analysis known as a morbidity-and-mortality (M&M) conference. Such conferences, reviewing how a patient has been treated, are a standard method by which medical and surgical services maintain standards of excellence.

In the Schiavo case, such an M&M assessment, considering all the factors at play in her treatment, would probably conclude that in the early years after her injury she had received first-rate care. She was carried through the acute phase, when she could easily have died. Having settled into a state of partial recovery, she was then taken to rehabilitative and physiotherapeutic centers for further assessment and treatment. There she was seen by several expert clinicians, started on intragastric feedings, and protected from infections of her pulmonary and urinary tract—all with the purpose of observing her neurological and psychological condition and hoping for further recovery.

When her trajectory of recovery leveled off, she was brought back to her neighborhood for care. Here, one phase gave way to another as what might be thought of as the rescue mission changed gradually into a sustaining mission, based on the realization that she was living with a brain injury unlikely to improve further and that what remained of her life would be spent in bed, in a limitedly responsive state. Bringing her into a hospice for the performance of this sustaining mission was another excellent clinical decision.

Hospice teams are made up of doctors, nurses, social workers, and physiotherapists who together develop a plan to care for someone in an incurable and usually terminal phase of life. In contrast to hospital services, hospice teams do not see time as being "of the essence." Of the essence now is, instead, the development of mutual understanding among all the parties—patient, family, and caregivers—concerning aims and actions suitable to helping the one who suffers. Achieving those goods usually *takes* time, for everything depends on gaining and retaining the family's confidence that the team really cares about the patient—is committed to doing its best to sustain what can be sustained, to alleviate suffering while at the same time not demanding heroic sacrifices from anyone.

This last point is very important. In a hospice, the staff does not provide a ventilator or cardiac monitoring at a patient's bedside—because there is no plan to transfer the patient to an acute treatment center for respiratory or cardiac support. But neither does the staff believe that, for patients with long-standing and incurable conditions, one can or should ignore the possibility of helping them live a less painful life, even if that might mean a shorter one. Thus, a hospice will treat the symptoms of certain potentially deadly conditions like bowel obstructions, cardiac arrhythmias, blood clots, and some infections but will not treat the conditions themselves.

In hospice care, no one is deprived of the simple amenities of being kept clean and receiving food and water. In Terri Schiavo's case, just as the team did not withdraw her bladder catheter, which helped keep her clean, so it did not withdraw the gastric tube, which had similarly been put in place during the rescue phase in order to ease the burden of nursing her. If for some reason the gastric tube had to be removed, the team would surely have tried to sustain nutrition by feeding her with spoon and cup.

In a hospice, decisions to limit medical services are made easier by everyone's knowledge of how the patient's condition emerged. Team attention, emphasizing as it does all relevant perspectives, strives to support all relevant interests. Terri Schiavo received good care and treatment and would not have been permitted to suffer unnecessarily. At the same time, she would not have been carried repeatedly through processes of treatment that ultimately did nothing to advance the quality of her life. Reasoning in a similar way and in full consciousness, Pope John Paul II elected not to return to a hospital for the third time in a month for treatment of his fatal condition. Instead, and despite the increased risks, he accepted the treatments available in his home.

The overarching principle that hospice doctors and nurses strive to represent and exemplify is never to betray a patient to death or act directly to kill. They may help a patient *surrender* to death, by forgoing active medical procedures when these provide nothing but empty time and extend the period of suffering. And their particular judgments in this regard may well be challenged as ambiguous—or even arbitrary—by those with a legal mind or an ax to grind. But those judgments are usually clear to everyone working in a hospice, just as the distinction between betrayal and surrender is clear in other situations in life.

It was in this phase of caring for Terri Schiavo that things went badly wrong. As we have seen, her husband had begun to despair for her and for his own future. As far as the public record shows, he seems to have been given little reason to rekindle his hopes. In particular, no functional studies (like an MRI) were done to determine whether her cerebral cortex, the brain region most responsible for coherent behavior, showed any evidence of recovering. Nor did the testimony of bedside observers help. While some thought they saw evidence of slow but tiny steps toward consciousness, others thought that she displayed only reflex reactions.

He was told her diagnosis was "persistent vegetative state." Predictably, this label complicated rather than aided the situation, encouraging those who thought that she no longer existed as an animate being and infuriating those who believed it labeled her a vegetable. That is precisely why most neuro-psychiatrists who work in hospices, even though they acknowledge the term's diagnostic accuracy, are reluctant to use it. Instead, they describe patients like Terri Schiavo in the language of neuropathology. Thus, they might have spoken of her as being in a "decorticate" condition, a term that not only indicates the problem but helps everyone—doctors, nurses, family members—think more dispassionately about how to evaluate it.

As these events unfolded, the plan of sustaining her in a hospice fell apart. Her guardian husband could no longer be persuaded to allow her to be fed, and under Florida law he had the right to demand that her nutrition be stopped. The courts were called in, and in the end judges and policemen removed the hospice team from her care, starving her until she died. No one was satisfied with the outcome. It came too slowly to suit her husband, and it came too brutally to comfort her parents. As for the hospice staff, so deeply biased in favor of sustaining life, one can only imagine their anguish.

So what, our imagined M&M conference leaders might ask, can one learn from this story? When I first considered this question along with several other doctors and nurses experienced in hospice care, we were nonplussed. Although we had treated hundreds of patients like Terri Schiavo, none of us had experienced a failure like this one. Our first thought was that other matters must have been at work—old resentments, unacknowledged jealousies, envy, bitter conflicts over money—to generate the kind of abuse of a patient so visible here. Only gradually, with publication of the reports, decisions, and interviews, did the explanation become clear.

As soon as Terri Schiavo's case moved into the law courts of Florida, the concept of "life under altered circumstances" went by the boards—and so, necessarily, did any consideration of how to serve such life. Both had been trumped by the concept of "life unworthy of life" and how to end it.

I use the term *life unworthy of life* advisedly. The phrase first appeared a long time ago—as the title of a book published in Germany in 1920, coauthored by a lawyer and a psychiatrist. *Die Freigabe der Vernichtung lebensunwertes Leben* translates as "Lifting Constraint from the Annihilation of Life Unworthy of Life." Terri Schiavo's husband and his clinical and legal advisers, believing that hers was now a life unworthy of life, sought, and achieved, its annihilation. Claiming to respect her undocumented wish not to live dependently, they were willing to have her suffer pain and, by specific force of law, to block her caregivers from offering her oral feedings of the kind provided to all terminal patients in a hospice—even to the point of prohibiting mouth-soothing ice chips. Everything else flowed from here.

How could such a thing happen? This, after all, is not Nazi Germany, where the culture of death foreshadowed in the awful title of that book would reach such horrendous public proportions. But we in this country have our own, home-grown culture of death, whose face is legal and moral and benignly individualistic rather than authoritarian and pseudoscientific. It has many roots, which would require a long historical treatise to unravel, with obligatory chapters considering such factors as the growth of life-sustaining and life-extending technologies and the dilemmas they bring, the increasingly assertive deprecation of medical expertise and understanding in favor of patients' "autonomous" decision making, the explosion in rights-related personal law and the associated explosion in medical-malpractice suits, and much else besides.

All this has resulted in a steady diminution in the bonds of implicit trust between patients and their doctors and its replacement, in some cases by suspicion or outright hostility, in many other cases by an almost reflexive unwillingness on the part of doctors to impose their own considered, prudential judgments—including their ethical judgments—on the course of treatment. In the meantime, a new discipline has stepped into the breach; its avowed purpose is to help doctors and patients alike reach decisions in difficult situations, and it is now a mandatory subject of study in medical and nursing schools.

I am speaking, of course, about bioethics, which came into being around the same time as the other developments I have been describing. To the early leaders of this discipline, it was plain that doctors and nurses, hitherto guided by professional codes of conduct and ancient ideals of virtue embedded in the Hippocratic oath or in the career and writings of Florence Nightingale, were in need of better and more up-to-date instruction. But, being theorists rather than medical practitioners, most bioethicists proved to be uninterested in developing the characters of doctors and nurses. Rather, they were preoccupied with identifying perceived conflicts between the "aims" of doctors and the "rights" of patients and with prescribing remedies for those conflicts.

Unlike in medicine itself, these remedies are untested and untestable. They have multiplied nevertheless, to the point where they have become fixtures in the lives of all of us, an unquestioned part of our vocabulary, subtly influencing our most basic attitudes toward sickness and health and, above all, our assumptions about how to prepare ourselves for death. The monuments to the bioethicists' principles include Do Not Resuscitate (DNR) orders, the euphemistically named Living Wills, and the legalization of physician-assisted suicide in the state of Oregon. These are not all the same thing, to be sure, and sophisticated arguments can be advanced for each of them; cumulatively, however, they are signposts of our own culture of death.

Hospital administrators are generally pleased with bioethicists and the rationalizations they provide for ceasing care of the helpless and the disabled. By the same token, their presence is generally shunned by doctors and nurses, whose medical and moral vocabulary draws from different sources and whose training and experience have disposed them in a different direction. To most doctors and nurses, in any case, the idea that one can control the manner and pace of one's dying is largely a fantasy. They have seen what they have seen, and what they know is that at the crucial moments in this process, no document on earth can substitute for the one-on-one judgment, fallible as it may ultimately be, of a sensible, humane, and experienced physician.

Contemporary bioethics has become a natural ally of the culture of death, but the culture of death itself is a perennial human temptation; for onlookers in particular, it offers a reassuring answer ("this is how X would have wanted it") to otherwise excruciating dilemmas, and it can be rationalized every which way till Sunday. In Terri Schiavo's case, it is what won out over the hospice's culture of life, overwhelming by legal means, and by the force of advanced social opinion, the moral and medical command to choose life, to comfort the afflicted, and to teach others how to do the same. The more this culture continues to influence our thinking, the deeper are likely to become the divisions within our society and within our families, the more hardened our hatreds, and the more manifold our fears. More of us will die prematurely; some of us will even be persuaded that we want to.

Commentary, 2005

Hippocrates à la Mode

The Hippocratic oath sets forth a number of ethical principles for medical practice. It does so in the classical Greek fashion: first stating the aim of the enterprise and then describing the ethical implications embedded in such an aim. In recent years, as I attended the annual graduation ceremonies at the Johns Hopkins School of Medicine and also at Harvard, I became aware that the version of the Hippocratic oath recited by the graduating students was changing and, in particular, that as the years passed its ethical prescriptions were phrased less sharply, more vaguely. That the ethical standards of physicians were becoming steadily more nebulous at a time when clinical standards were becoming steadily more precise seemed an odd, ironic evolution.

Oaths are not directives—such as the Ten Commandments. They reflect how the takers of an oath are trying to behave. Indeed, they are attempts to make explicit on solemn occasions those ideals honored implicitly in daily life. They thus depict an ethos as much as they define a tenet. Nonetheless, oaths should point to specific actions that spring from clear principles. But on Commencement Day, vague sentiment seemed to prevail, and I began to ask why.

As it turned out, I was listening to an oath at Hopkins that was evolving. A recitation of the Hippocratic oath had not been part of the Hopkins graduating traditions until the late 1960s, when the students asked that it be included so as to give solemnity to what they perceived as an arid ceremony at a milestone in their lives. They consulted Professor Owsei Temkin, then director of the Institute of the History of Medicine at Hopkins, to identify a suitable translation for them, which he did—though with some reservations because oath taking did not appeal to him. He thought that oath takers seldom understood what they were saying and usually, perhaps fortunately, forgot all about it later. Nevertheless, in 1968, the graduating class rose and recited this translation of the Hippocratic oath (table 1) (Edelstein, 1967, p. 6) minus the invocation of pagan gods and lifetime family partnership with teachers.

It produced an uproar—not from the students but from members of the faculty dismayed by the abortion clause ("I will not give to a woman an abortive remedy"). All subsequent recitations by later classes removed that clause along with the admonition against "the knife" because, quite obviously, future surgeons as well as future internists were graduating. These initial alterations, however, launched a custom of amending the oath over time, and it was the later changes that caught my attention. But to appreciate their significance, a close look at the original is necessary.

The Hippocratic oath is divided into four parts. In the first, the gods and goddesses are evoked to witness the oath taking. The second

---

TABLE 1

The Hippocratic Oath

I.

"I swear by Apollo Physician and Asclepius and Hygieia and Panaceia and all the gods and goddesses, making them my witnesses, that I will fulfill according to my ability and judgment this oath and this covenant:

II.

To hold him who has taught me this art as equal to my parents and to live my life in partnership with him, and if he is in need of money to give him a share of mine, and to regard his offspring as equal to my brothers in male lineage and to teach them this art—if they desire to learn it—without fee and covenant; to give a share of precepts and oral instruction and all the other learning to my sons and to the sons of him who has instructed me and to pupils who have signed the covenant and have taken an oath according to the medical law, but to no one else.

IIIa.

I will apply dietetic measures for the benefit of the sick according to my ability and judgment, I will keep them from harm and injustice.

I will neither give a deadly drug to anybody if asked for it, nor will I make a suggestion to this effect. Similarly I will not give to a woman an abortive remedy. In purity and holiness I will guard my life and my art.

I will not use the knife, not even on sufferers from stone, but will withdraw in favor of such men as are engaged in this work.

IIIb.

Whatever houses I may visit, I will come for the benefit of the sick, remaining free of all intentional injustice, of all mischief and in particular of sexual relations with both female and male persons, be they free or slaves.

What I may see or hear in the course of the treatment or even outside of the treatment in regard to the life of men, which on no account one must spread abroad, I will keep to myself holding such things shameful to be spoken about.

IV.

If I fulfill this oath and do not violate it, may it be granted to me to enjoy life and art, being honored with fame among all men for all time to come; if I transgress it and swear falsely, may the opposite of all this be my lot."

is a long acknowledgment of the gratitude students entering into the practice of medicine feel toward those who teach them. The third, and key, part has two sections. In each the goal of medical practice is specified in the first sentence as: "I will [act] for the benefit of the sick." Then the goal is delineated by identifying a number of behaviors that support or oppose this aim. These Hippocratic ethical prescriptions render the meaning of "benefiting" the sick explicit. The prescriptions include admonitions against going beyond one's professional skills—that is what withdrawing in favor of the surgeon means—and against taking sexual advantage of patients or members of their household. The Greeks are nothing if not specific as they define the several sexual partners a physician might find in a household he visited. The oath closes by decreeing bleak consequences on doctors who fail to live as promised. Note the classic structure—a goal of action is identified and then the constitutive, inherent ethical implications flowing from this goal are prescribed.

TABLE 2

The Hippocratic Oath: The Johns Hopkins's Versions

1985 version	*1994 version*
"I do solemnly swear . . . by that which I hold most sacred . . . That I will be loyal to the profession of medicine . . . and just and generous to its members . . . That I will lead my life . . . and practice my art . . . in uprightness and honor . . . That into whatsoever house I shall enter . . . it shall be for the good of the sick . . . to the utmost of my power . . . holding myself aloof from wrong . . . from corruption . . . and from the tempting of others to vice . . . That I will exercise my art . . . solely for the care of my patients . . . and will give no drug . . . and perform no operation . . . for a *criminal purpose* . . . far less suggest it . . . That whatsoever I shall see or hear . . . of the lives of *men* . . . which is not fitting to be spoken . . . I will keep inviolably secret . . . These things I do promise . . . and in proportion as I am faithful to this my oath . . . may happiness and good repute be ever mine . . . the opposite if I shall be forsworn."	"I do solemnly swear . . . by that which I hold most sacred . . . That I will be loyal to the profession of medicine . . . and just in my relationships with its members . . . That I will lead my life . . . and practice my art . . . in uprightness and honor . . . That into whatsoever house I shall enter . . . it shall be for the good of the sick . . . to the utmost of my power . . . holding myself aloof from wrong . . . from corruption . . . and from the tempting of others to vice . . . That I will exercise my art . . . solely for the care of my patients . . . and will give no drug . . . and perform no operation . . . *without justifiable purpose* . . . far less suggest it . . . That whatsoever I shall see or hear . . . of the lives of *men and women* . . . which is not fitting to be spoken . . . I will keep inviolably secret . . . These things I do promise . . . and in proportion as I am faithful to this my oath . . . may happiness and good repute be ever mine . . . the opposite if I shall be forsworn."

Note: Ellipses represent pauses in the recitation of the oath.

Now look at the 1985 and 1994 Johns Hopkins versions of the Hippocratic oath (table 2). They resemble the original. Similar expressions certainly appear. These include acting "for the good of the sick." Although the abortion and "knife" clauses are gone, the contemporary meaning of "vice" as sexual immorality is employed, rephrasing the Greek specifications against sexual exploitation. The oath is shorter because the roster of gods and goddesses is omitted and the number of promises to fellow practitioners reduced.

But something is lost—a certain tough-mindedness. Indeed, although the Hippocratic goal—to benefit the sick—remains, it is not the first assertion about behavior. Rather, the expression "I will lead my life and practice my art in uprightness and honor" leads off. Not a bad sentiment certainly, but hardly one restricted to physicians or one from which specific behavioral admonitions flow. In fact, what follows at Hopkins has a much looser organization than the original. And on reflection, the initial comment smacks, if ever so slightly, of self-absorption—a modern fault.

An even closer reading of these two Hopkins versions reveals more of this unfortunate self-interest. Notice that in 1985 the Hopkins graduates swear that in their loyalty to the profession of medicine they will be "just and generous to its members." In 1994 they promise only to be "just." What happened to generous?! Again in 1985 the doctors say they will perform "no operation for a criminal purpose," but then in 1994 they state they will perform "no operation without justifiable purpose." That's a big change from Hippocrates. Certainly in this century, physicians have justified actions that no one could conceive of as "benefiting the sick." Finally, in 1994 the students promised to keep secret aspects of the lives of men and women. Not simply men as in 1985—a step forward in what otherwise I take to be a devolution of Hippocrates.

What was happening at Hopkins was not unique, as I soon discovered. In fact, the oaths now taken on graduation from Harvard Medical School provide a still better glimpse of the ethos behind contemporary medical ethics (Hupert, 1994, pp. 42–44). The students at Harvard decided—I'm sure wisely—that bowdlerizing the Hippocratic oath has problems. Therefore they wrote their own "Graduate Oath" that, again, has had several versions (table 3). By comparing these two versions one can grasp not only the ethos from which these newly minted doctors emerge but also the specific actions they see as important enough to encourage.

They also express nice sentiments, some of which resemble ideas in the Hippocratic oath. However, the Harvard oaths are even more ambiguous than the Hopkins versions and enlarge the commitment to self-interest.

The Harvard authors abandon precision right at the start when they replace the Hippocratic aim—the benefit of the sick—with "the service of humanity." As a goal, the service of humanity not only is more imprecise but also may occasionally conflict with "the benefit

---

TABLE 3

The Graduate Oath: Harvard's Versions

1989 version	*1994 version*
"Now being admitted to the profession of medicine/dentistry, I solemnly pledge to use my skills in the service of humanity. I recognize an obligation to serve my patients, my profession and my community. I will serve all in need without bias and with openness of spirit. The health and quality of life of my patient will be my first consideration. I will hold in confidence all that my patient entrusts to me. I will strive to promote honor within the medical/dental profession. My colleagues will be as my family. I will give to my teachers and to my students the respect and gratitude which is their due. *I will maintain the utmost respect for human life. Even under threat, I will not use my knowledge contrary to the laws of humanity.* I will promote the health and welfare of my community. *To serve others most effectively, I must maintain my own well-being.* Today I will seek to discover my errors of yesterday, and tomorrow I will strive to obtain new light on what I am sure of today. I will seek the opportunity for personal fulfillment in my role as a physician/dentist. These promises I make freely and upon my honor."	"Now being admitted to the profession of medicine/dentistry, I pledge myself to the service of humanity. I recognize my obligation to serve my patients, my community and my profession. I will use my skills to serve all in need, with openness of spirit and without bias. The health and well-being of my patients will be my first consideration. I will hold in confidence all that my patients entrust to me. *I will not subordinate the dignity of any person to scientific or political ends. I recognize that I have responsibilities to my community: to promote its welfare and to speak out against injustice. The high regard of my profession is born of society's trust in its practitioners;* I will strive to merit that trust. I will promote the integrity of my profession through honest and respectful relations with fellow health professionals. I am indebted to those who have taught me the art and science of my profession and I recognize my responsibility, in turn, to contribute to the humane education of future doctors. I will strive to advance my profession by seeking new knowledge and by reexamining the ideas and practices of the past. *I assume these responsibilities knowing that their fulfillment depends upon my own good health. I ask that my colleagues be attentive to my well-being, as I will be to theirs.* I will seek to improve my practice by addressing my mistakes and maintaining my skills. I take this oath freely and upon my honor."

Note: Italic added.

of the sick," particularly if sick people are identified as burdens. For example, the Nazi doctors (Burleigh, 1994, p. 275), the zealots for euthanasia, and the Tuskegee scientists (who withheld treatment to observe the "natural history" of syphilitic infection) claimed that they intended to provide some service for humanity through their actions.

Because the "service of humanity" is so abstract and nondiscriminating, the ethical principles that follow in the Harvard oaths lack the steel of definite purpose. In fact, there are few limits to what the writers can propose. Thus they claim that "the health and quality of life ["well-being" in the second version] of my patient will be my first consideration"—thus provoking a concern for their second or third considerations. These emerge in lofty language as vague promises to ambiguous entities such as "the community," "the society," and "the profession." The oath breaks up into fragmentary bits and pieces of worthy impulses, residues of other unstated goals and intentions—some quite remote from medical practice.

Indeed, a new and farcically self-centered tenet emerges briefly in 1989 to be enhanced in 1994. On its first appearance, the authors write, "To serve others most effectively, I must maintain my own well-being"—a sentiment suitable for a bodybuilder. In 1994 they carry this impulse further, saying, "I assume these responsibilities knowing that their fulfillment depends upon my own good health. I ask that my colleagues be attentive to my well-being, as I will be to theirs." Am I alone in hearing a smug self-absorption in these words? Did not others at Harvard detect the contemporary faddish worship of health so prone to forget that for some things—such as freedom and the care of the sick—health must occasionally be risked, indeed even sacrificed? Such articulations of ethics à la mode are all about benefits to the physician and only remotely about "benefit to the sick." If these sentences accurately represent opinions of recent Harvard Medical School graduates, they must have absorbed the ethos of "me" that the witty American author Tom Wolfe (Wolfe, 1976) described enveloping us all.

More troublesome (and less amusing than this parsimonious concern over the one feature youth has in lieu of experience—vigorous health) is what was omitted when the 1994 version replaced that of 1989. Paragraph 4 of the 1989 version reflects the Hippocratic source of some of its sentiments by saying, "I will maintain the utmost respect for human life. Even under threat, I will not use my knowledge contrary to the laws of humanity." These sentences are dropped from the oath of 1994. They are replaced with "I will not subordinate the dignity of any person to scientific or political ends" (that dignity is more important than life is a novel medical idea) and by "I recognize that I have responsibilities to my community: to promote its welfare and to speak out against injustice. The high regard of my profession is born of society's trust in its practitioners; I will strive to merit that trust." Surely society's trust in physicians rests upon knowing that doctors have proved ready—often at great personal hazard—to battle "for the benefit of the sick" and to prevail by enhancing diagnosis, treatment, and prevention of disease. Everybody must fight injustice; doctors fight disease.

What do I conclude? That the best and brightest young doctors recite such self-serving and jejune oaths is more than an embarrassment. It's a false step at a time of great vulnerability for medicine, a time when others such as "health" managers and government legislators are ready to define—with clarity—just what doctors will do.

Professor Temkin was right. If this is the outcome, medical students should stop reciting—and certainly stop writing—oaths. They are so confused about their ethical aims, so mixed up in the sources of their ideals, that they should stop talking about them in public. They would do better to proceed in the service of the sick and so discover, during their quest to do that well, the ideals underlying the practice of medicine.

In that quest they will learn much about themselves as they respond to the demands—physical, intellectual, moral—intrinsic to medical service. They will also come to realize how many forces outside the medical profession—commercial, bureaucratic, ideological—must be resisted in order to protect the life and morale of sick people today. If the students are reflective, they will eventually perceive that nothing they gleaned in these trials would have surprised Hippocrates (Temkin, 1991). *Nature Medicine*, 1996

REFERENCES

Burleigh, M. (1994). *Death and deliverance: "Euthanasia" in Germany, 1900–1945.* Cambridge: Cambridge University Press.

Edelstein, L. (1967). *Ancient medicine.* Ed. O. Temkin and C. L. Temkin. Baltimore: Johns Hopkins Press.

Hupert, N. (1994). What's in an oath? *Harvard Medical Alumni Bulletin* 68 (2): 42–44.

Temkin, O. (1991). *Hippocrates in a world of pagans and Christians.* Baltimore: Johns Hopkins University Press.

Wolfe, T. (1976). The me decade and the third great awakening. In *Mauve gloves and madmen, clutter and vine,* 111–147. New York: Farrar, Straus, and Giroux.

Part III

A WOEFUL MISDIRECTION
OF A TRADITION

Paul Roazen was the first to point out that we should not speak of Freud's "discoveries"—as though he had found something comparable to the discoveries of Galileo or Mendel—but rather speak of Freud's conceptions and the power they had in their time. Freud did not "discover" the unconscious but proposed a concept of it as built by repression and organized around libidinal conflicts. He proposed a theory of infantile sexuality as the provocative source of these conflicts and explained their repression by parental oversight. His treatment setting with its "couch" and its method of free association seemed new but derived some of its authority from its resemblance to the methods of the mesmeric healers and hypnotists of his time. Most important, he conceived a worldview and drew many followers into a powerful movement of support for that worldview in which the initiates to his ideas might see deeply into human mental life.

Freud was a genius—of narrative description, of coherent prose argument, of organization, of self-promotion. In his work he developed such an internally coherent theoretical system that those who became embedded within it sometimes lost any infrastructure with which to reason outside the system. With experience, however, they often became coherent and friendly sources of support for their patients and came to understand them and some of the difficulties they faced. They frequently did much good and caring work in the clinic even as their worldview probably retarded the growth of the culture at large.

I soon learned, however, that many contemporary psychotherapists—who often see themselves as "reformers" of Freud and sometimes as advocates for one of his contemporaries, Pierre Janet—are poor copies of the master and have been vulnerable to being swept up in fads which identify other provocative sources of unconscious conflict and repression. I call them the "manneristic Freudians": they copy the master's style but lack the master's genius. Not only did they lack the generosity and kindness that the orthodox Freudians retained as they matured, but they often became wild protagonists for a revisionist history of Freud's work (claiming that he cowardly did not face down his critics of his first ideas)—a revisionist history that launched the memory wars of the late 1980s and early 1990s.

I was drawn into these wars, and the essays in this section give some sense of them and the many distressing aspects of the results. Freud's "worldview" must take some blame for the wars, but most of the orthodox Freudian psychiatrists whom I came to meet in these wars were fervent critics of the ideologues. I think that the main battles have been won but occasional skirmishes still break out, all giving credence to the idea that this was a public craze that now is in a dormant phase but could break into flame if the lessons here are not fully appreciated.

The Death of Freud and
the Rebirth of Psychiatry

The condition of psychiatry today can be compared to that of Russia after the fall of communism. Like Russia after Marxism, psychiatry after Freudianism has lost its once dominant doctrine. Like that vast nation attempting to operate under a rudimentary capitalism, psychiatry now labors under the sway of a classificatory system, the *Diagnostic and Statistical Manual of Mental Disorders* (DSM-IV), so crude as to foster inept educational programs and clumsy clinical practices. Just as Russia searches for a structure to replace communism, so psychiatry, with Freudianism in ruins, struggles to find a coherent concept of the mental disorders and the best way to treat them.

Surveying this confusing scene, the anthropologist T. M. Luhrmann has produced *Of Two Minds: The Growing Disorder in American Psychiatry* (2000), a bleak assessment of contemporary psychiatric education. Casting her eye on the "enculturation" of young psychiatrists into their profession, she argues that the recent discoveries in biomedicine, which the public may think are great advances, have in fact plucked the "soul" from psychiatry, leaving it a cold business that dispenses magical pills rather than addressing patients in all their tragic particularity.

Much of Luhrmann's criticism is dead-on, and it is useful to have it said in this public way. Unfortunately, she concludes that the answer is a return to Freudian psychoanalysis. It is as though, after visiting Russia, an anthropologist decided the country had made an enormous mistake in abandoning Marxism. Luhrmann misleads for two reasons: she slights the history of psychiatry, aspects of which explain both its problems and its promise; and, more important, she neglects fundamental issues of method—particularly those of assessing, differentiating, and understanding patients—from which therapeutics emerge. Thus, Luhrmann fails to see that the present, with all its shortcomings, is actually auspicious, a stage in the development of psychiatry in which, even amid the rubble, it is possible to discern the foundations of progress.

I began my own career in psychiatry in the 1950s, in the middle of what historian Edward Shorter called "the hiatus," the generation-long period, roughly from 1935 to 1975, when Freudianism was the unchallenged doctrine of American psychiatry. During the hiatus, psychiatry ceased to grow as a science-based, evidence-driven discipline.

As medical students, my classmates and I were taught that psychoanalysis had revealed that mental disorders differed only in degree, not in kind. Mental disorders were invariably the consequences of mishandled early-life conflicts of a sexual nature—universal experiences varying in severity. We were taught that particular symptoms identified the character of those conflicts; no other evidence was needed because the "symptoms tell the tale." Compulsiveness and perfectionism denoted overforceful toilet training in infancy, anxiety was the product of the childhood discovery of anatomical differences between boys and girls, and paranoid suspicions gave evidence of repressed homosexual conflict.

We were also taught that these early conflicts and pathogenic events were masked by repression but alive in the "dynamic" unconscious, shaping our mental life. Because sexual conflicts in infancy were universal, no real distinction existed between us students and the patients. We were taught that if our society altered its methods of child rearing and attitudes toward sex, mental disorder would diminish and all would be well. A brave new world seemed to be dawning.

At the same time, we students noted that the psychiatric wards differed radically from other medical wards, like neurology, cardiology, and surgery. The most obvious difference was that on the psychiatric wards not only the patients but most of the staff were in therapy. Again, this practice was prompted by the theory that psychiatrists and patients differed only in degree of disorder. Young psychiatrists were told to think of themselves as "little messes" caring for "bigger messes." Their supervisors encouraged this idea.

With most doctors, nurses, social workers, and even office personnel in therapy, the libidinal minidramas of everyone's encounters with his or her therapist became a topic of gossip within psychiatric centers. Certain psychoanalysts (particularly those who claimed close descent from Freud and retained the accents of old Vienna) dominated these centers and frequently used the political power that came from knowing many secrets to advance their favorites and banish their foes.

The psychiatrists-in-training, preoccupied by their own therapy, gravitated toward the patients who were most like themselves, withdrawing attention from the seriously mentally ill (patients with schizophrenia and manic-depression). Young and articulate patients, often female and worried over romantic adversities, were sought out, especially if they (or their parents) were wealthy enough to support the standard psychoanalytic treatment, a years-long course of fifty-minute therapy sessions as frequent as five times a week. A corrupting self-absorption pervaded psychiatric departments.

The seriously mentally ill—the counterparts of the seriously physically ill, who were the mainstays of training programs in the other medical specialties—were considered "too regressed" for educational purposes, too damaged by experience in their childhood to be promptly helped by psychotherapy. They were transferred to the state hospitals, though authorities in the universities promised that their time for treatment would come after the less seriously disturbed had resolved their troubles. It never did.

Scientific research was neglected. Why do research when we already knew, on the basis of Freud's writings, just what constituted the causes of mental problems? Research—if you can dignify such work by that term—took the form of composing ingenious metaphors linking conjectured sexual conflicts to the symptoms seen in patients.

The classic Freudian example proposed that paranoid delusions—especially the persecutory, jealous, or amorous ones—were all distorted expressions of homosexual conflict derived from "arrests" in childhood sexual development. Thus a man's latent, unconscious, and unacceptable idea "I love him," once transformed by unconscious mechanisms, manifested itself as one of three delusional beliefs: the persecutory ("He hates me"), the jealous ("My wife loves him"), or the amorous ("Another woman loves me").

By the 1950s, leading American psychoanalysts were competing to see who could derive the flashiest connections from superficial resemblances between mental symptoms and events in patients' lives. The interpretation of genital symbols became a way of finding sexual meaning in mental disorders. None of this could be called research, and none of it advanced the care and treatment of patients or the elucidation of mental illnesses.

A telling and ultimately fatal flaw within the psychoanalytic movement was its fissiparous character—present almost from the start, when Adler and Jung split from Freud to produce their own schools of thought. In America, the Freudian school was initially successful in dominating the strategically crucial centers of the university clinics and teaching hospitals in the East and the salons of Los Angeles and Hollywood in the West (where Freudian ideas influenced the motion picture industry).

Dissension between orthodox and reform sects of American Freudianism soon erupted, as subgroups of psychoanalysts hived off into separate psychoanalytic training institutes in every large city, with much ill will and repudiation all round. Each center devolved its own organization, initiation rights, rules of membership, and official doctrine about the "keys to meaning." Each presented itself as providing a different kind of analyst—and postulants faced the problem of choosing among them. This fractionalizing demonstrated the cultic character of psychoanalysis; it was more Greco-Roman than modern in its call for commitments to different conceptions of reality rather than to the single medico-scientific method guided by observation, reason, and experiment.

This sectarianism not only added heat to psychoanalytic convictions but also made criticism of Freudian ideas more difficult. Psychoanalytic propositions became moving targets, and challenges from psychiatrists outside the establishment were evaded or rejected as ignorant of the present state of the art.

I can testify to the frustration felt by those questioning psychoanalytic concepts such as repression, the dynamic unconscious, dream interpretation, and the rest of it. We were dismissed as being either in bad faith ("Freud bashing") or simple-minded and insensitive, given the "advancing" character of theory and the subtle, "concerned" thought of psychoanalysts. I learned firsthand the validity of philosopher Ernest Gellner's comment about psychoanalysis: "Evasion is not brought in to save the theory: It is the theory."

During the 1960s, events conspired to bring the dominance of psychoanalysis in America to a end. The most dramatic of these was deinstitutionalization of the seriously mentally ill. This radical venture rested on two related justifications. The chief one came from the discovery (mostly by chance) in the 1950s and 1960s of medicines that acted against the symptoms of schizophrenia and manic-depression, relieving the hallucinations and delusions that had kept patients sequestered in mental hospitals. It was only logical that the mentally ill—who, remember, in theory were just like the rest of us only more seriously disturbed—shouldn't be locked up in distant hospitals if medications could make them less threatening and dangerous. They deserved what the less ill had long been allowed: freedom to look after themselves, while receiving psychotherapy in centers for ambulatory patients.

Vast deinstitutionalization of the mentally ill was launched in the late 1960s. Patients who had lived for years in outlying, dilapidated state psychiatric hospitals were released to urban and academic psychiatric centers for treatment. The psychiatrists there, previously honored for their therapeutic skills, found that they could not manage these new arrivals. They did not understand the medications that had been used in the state hospitals, and the Freudian-based psychotherapies, so time-consuming, were ineffective. The patients spilled out into the city streets, and the deficiencies of psychiatric know-how became obvious to anyone with open eyes.

The psychopharmacological advances on which these hospital discharges depended also made it possible to differentiate patients. How could anyone claim that mental illness is all one, à la Freudianism, when only patients with manic excitement responded to lithium salts? And if antidepressant and antischizophrenic medications worked only for certain patients, then one must conclude that the patients differed in their brains. As distinctions like these became critical for treatment, psychiatrists began to look back to the decades around the turn of the century when the distinctions between conditions such as manic-depression and schizophrenia had first been identified.

Psychiatry began to stumble toward the path of empirical science that general medicine had followed since the mid-nineteenth century. Progress began to appear, especially in the diagnosis and treatment of the seriously ill. Psychotherapy itself came under study, and several investigative psychiatrists began to challenge the claim that cure came from treating the Freudian "pathogenic" events of childhood— the Oedipal complex, castration anxiety, penis envy, and the like.

Dr. Jerome Frank at Johns Hopkins, a pioneer in psychotherapy research, investigated hundreds of patients and concluded that healing depended upon general rather than specific factors: the patient's receiving an acceptable and persuasive explanation for his or her distress from a therapist who could evoke some emotional arousal during the treatment and who carried some culturally licensed authority as a healer. These characteristics were common to many psychotherapies, not restricted to psychoanalytic ones.

More important, Frank proved that patients in psychotherapy did not resemble one another in the cause of their distress. No common theme of childhood sexual conflict or developmental arrest, no particular psychic complex, characterized them. Rather, these patients were alike in their symptoms and in the habitual ways they approached difficulties: they were all "demoralized," overmastered by some problem usually related to their present life. Frank noted that successful symptom-relieving psychotherapy worked by providing patients with ways to achieve mastery of their situations; it did not depend primarily on insight into early life conflicts. He demonstrated these facts about psychotherapy with standard scientific methods, among them placebo controls, comparative outcome studies, and numerate evidence.

Jerome Frank's work was an enormous challenge to both the theories and the practices of psychoanalysis. In the 1970s, Dr. Aaron T. Beck of the University of Pennsylvania furthered this advance in psychiatry by developing and teaching an effective psychotherapy that attempted to correct the self-defeating attitudes and assumptions that provoke demoralization. Calling his program "Cognitive Behavioral Therapy," he demonstrated in therapeutic trials that patients so treated recovered more frequently from depression and anxiety than did patients treated less systematically. Evidence-based psychotherapy at last became a reality.

Like Frank, Beck showed that no single attitude and no common early childhood trauma afflicted his patients. They all needed and responded to a treatment that uncovered how they were demoralized by their habitual attitudes and presumptions. These could be directly challenged and rescripted as the patient came to see the role they played in his or her distress and as the psychotherapist proposed and reinforced more constructive ways of thinking and responding to the circumstances life had set before the patient. Since Beck's work, other therapists have demonstrated ways of encouraging patients to recognize how their attitudes and assumptions are self-defeating and can be changed.

The preeminence of Freudian psychoanalysis was essentially over by the end of the 1970s. Freudianism did not end with a bang, as did Marxism. It just petered out, as fewer and fewer of the best students came to believe that they should devote time to it—though a nostalgia for psychoanalysis persists in some circles to this day.

T. M. Luhrmann's *Of Two Minds* turns out to be just such a nostalgic glance back. Begun as an empirical work, it is the product of her four-year study of American psychiatric education. Luhrmann—a professor at the University of California–San Diego and author of previous works on ritual magic and colonial society—visited a number of centers where psychiatrists are trained. She observed the care being delivered by resident psychiatrists and the teaching methods employed to guide them. She put in long hours talking with teachers, residents, medical students, and patients.

In many of the centers she visited, Luhrmann found confusion and misdirection. Sometimes she found students deeply distressed over conflicts among their teachers and over the restrictions placed on services by insurers. She reveals how, in some training centers, the teaching of thoughtless diagnostic formulas and reflexive prescriptions for medication is dehumanizing the contacts between patients and psychiatrists. Depression? Bring out the Prozac. Attention deficit disorder? Toss down the Ritalin. The very advances in biomedicine that have immensely facilitated the treatment of mental illness have damaged the psychiatric profession. Young psychiatrists lack both the time and the interest to bring their patients "the commitment we feel toward full-fledged human beings."

But a problem arises. Early in her book, Luhrmann notes that, in preparation for her immersion in the field of psychiatry, she herself entered into psychoanalytic psychotherapy. She did so because psychoanalysts told her that, if she were a patient with them, her understanding of the educational and treatment services she would be witnessing would be deepened. Unfortunately, her own psychoanalysis has left her a partisan, a captive of one of the vested interests whose influence on the course and content of psychiatric education she intended to study.

Because of this bias, Luhrmann found only in the outpatient services, where psychotherapy is dispensed, what she deemed a proper concern for individual patients. The title of her book, *Of Two Minds*, is intended to emphasize that students of psychiatry feel themselves citizens of two worlds: one of brain material and medications, the other of human feeling and the "soul-craft" of dynamic psychotherapy; one of white-coated scientists who expound on brain systems and medications and treat patients like objects, the other of thoughtful, tweed-coated psychotherapists explaining the tortured lives of people who, but for the grace of God, are you and I. Ominously weighing in on the side of the white coats are the administrators of managed care, who, Luhrmann says, see the soul-craft of psychotherapy as unnecessary.

Luhrmann champions psychoanalytic teaching as fundamental to the training of young psychiatrists. In this, she is simply mistaken. We can no more return to the old orthodoxy than Russia can revive the Soviet Union. Luhrmann fails to appreciate that psychiatry is well free of the dominance of a conjectural theory that cheated many patients out of helpful treatment and caused a great many talented students to waste years of their lives on fruitless study.

It may be that Luhrmann expects some compromise to emerge, in which a portion of the old Freudian creed is reassumed. Reasonable though this sounds, no middle ground is possible. The psychoanalyst and the science-based psychiatrist are not to be thought of as simply having different ways of interpreting an agreed-upon set of clinical observations—interpretations that could be negotiated between them. The hard fact is that the two take opposing positions over what *exists*—what counts as real in mental life—and how one should study it. Repudiation of the other, not conciliation, is the aim of each, as both parties will gladly explain.

I disagree with Luhrmann, too, about the role of managed care. Like many of the psychiatrists she talked with in her travels, she views it as menacing the future of psychiatric practice and education. But managed care, while an annoying burden, is one, I'm afraid, that psychiatrists brought on themselves. Back when psychological treatments ran solely on Freudian concepts, patients were often kept in treatment until their money ran out.

Little or no effort was made to test the efficacy of psychoanalytic programs. For all that the business ethic of managed care now threatens benefits to patients, this threat will subside when outcome studies demonstrate what evidence-based psychiatry can do. Psychiatrists must show how their diagnostic formulations and therapeutic plans lead to recoveries. Only then will they become powerful advocates for their patients and see their opinions taken seriously by health systems.

Where T. M. Luhrmann sees growing disorder in psychiatry, I see growing pains. These will be resolved through study of the methods that psychiatry uses, which Luhrmann neglects. Psychiatrists must learn how to think about different psychiatric patients. They must employ different methods of reasoning for different patients—methods that, though distinct in their application, are not in conflict.

The German psychiatrist and philosopher Karl Jaspers spoke to the fundamental issue of method with great penetration and lucidity in his magisterial book *General Psychopathology*, published in 1913. (Although brought out in English by the University of Chicago in 1963, this work has been largely unnoticed in the United States. It was reissued by the Johns Hopkins University Press in 1997.) Jaspers laid out the methods that psychiatrists need to employ to evaluate and make sense of the different mental disorders. He provided the rules, standards, and means for making useful, replicable observations of psychiatric patients. He delineated the different mental states and symptoms psychiatrists would find when they studied their patients systematically. And then he described the two distinct methods of reasoning available to psychiatrists to explain their patients' signs and symptoms.

Jaspers noted that psychiatrists, in seeking to explain mental illnesses, drew both from medical science, where the processes of nature that damage health are discerned, and from history, where fateful events and personal choices disrupt mental serenity. Specifically, he taught that some mental disorders derive from brain diseases whereas others derive from conflict between a person's hopes and what life deals out to him or her. He defined the strengths and limitations of each of these methods of reasoning: scientific reasoning from empirical evidence, and historical reasoning enriched by empathetic insight. He demonstrated how both are indispensable to the psychiatrist, who must not confuse one with the other.

By distinguishing the explanation offered by science from the compassionate understanding offered by history, Jaspers identified the epistemological and therapeutic divide into which Luhrmann stumbles. Jaspers proposed that psychiatrists receive an education in theory and practice demonstrating both methods in action—an education best provided by teachers who apply them in research. He wrote brilliantly about psychotherapy and also anticipated the advances in brain science and pharmacology we are witnessing today.

Jaspers saw not Luhrmann's two minds but a single psychiatry encompassing two explanatory methods. These methods are not difficult for a single mind to grasp if they are exemplified in teaching and research. They are readily integrated in practice—both for seriously ill patients who have major brain diseases and for demoralized patients facing conflicts in their personal lives.

But woe, Jaspers said, to those who do not understand the distinctions between these methods of reasoning and try to make one method dominate psychiatry. They will interrupt progress and alienate their students. Jaspers went unheeded in America, even as he warned against the tragically wasteful hiatus produced by Freudian dominance, which has left psychiatry today in its conceptually primitive state.

But I am optimistic. As psychiatry becomes more coherent—pushed in part by managed care and instructed in part by a reassessment of its methods of thought—psychiatrists can present themselves to the public just as physicians and surgeons do, and no longer as practitioners of a mystery cult, condescendingly proposing crude, sexualized ideas about human nature. Psychiatrists can then emerge as members of a medical specialty who, like all other doctors, are committed to healing—rather than indoctrinating—their patients.

The Weekly Standard, 2000

The End of a Delusion

The Psychiatric Memory Wars Are Over

At the end of the nineteenth century, Sigmund Freud—ever anxious to present an overarching, universal explanation for mental unrest—suggested that "repressed memories" of childhood sexual abuse are a common cause of adult mental disorders.

He quickly abandoned the idea (replacing it with the concept of infantile sexuality) when he saw that it harmed rather than helped his patients. But such ideas seem to have lives of their own, and a hundred years after Freud first proposed it, the idea of repressed memories rose again in new and even gaudier clothing. Grown beyond Freud's unadorned view of domestic misconduct, it came to include beliefs that many of these sexual traumas—which the troubled patients' shocked minds had repressed—took place during satanic rituals and experiments aboard alien spacecraft.

It is today almost impossible to understand how anyone ever believed this absurd and ridiculous notion, but it was less than a decade ago that the idea was flourishing in America. The American psychiatric and psychological establishment bears a shame that will be hard ever to wash away. Thousands of patients—thousands of sick, damaged people who had come to medical professionals for help—were destructively misdirected into trolling through their past in search of hidden sexual trauma. By the late 1980s, wards and clinics in university psychiatric departments, eminent hospitals, and even the National Institute of Mental Health were devoted to uncovering these repressed memories.

The craze for this psychiatric madness was never universal, and, to their credit, some theorists and practicing psychiatrists resisted the practices and ideas in what Frederick Crews aptly dubbed the "memory wars." The importance of Richard J. McNally's new book *Remembering Trauma* (2003) lies not just in the superb and definitive survey McNally makes of the history of repressed memories but also in what the book stands for: *Remembering Trauma* is the monument built to mark the end of the memory wars. The repressed-memory diagnosis has finally been repressed.

When these wars started, orthodox Freudianism—the concepts of psychoanalysis based on infantile sexuality and the dynamic unconscious that Freud developed on abandoning his child abuse idea— was losing influence after dominating psychiatric thought for more than two generations in America. The Freudian explanation and treatment were weak in practice, whatever their intrinsic intellectual interest. New and simpler treatments of psychiatric patients, as with medication and cognitive counseling, were emerging to replace it.

The idea of repressed memories was in many ways *anti*-Freudian, anathema to the orthodox Freudian view. But the explosion of interest in repressed memories was nonetheless a result of Freudianism— a notion born from the Freudian movement's death throes, something we might have anticipated had we reflected on the situation faced by therapists accustomed for so long to remarkable social and professional standing in America as keepers of the deep secrets of our minds.

More clamor about the Oedipus complex, castration anxiety, penis envy, and all the rest of the classic Freudian elements was not going to revive attention and energy for the sect. New kinds of secrets about human mental life and its disorders were needed. And what better than the idea that our parents—particularly our fathers—betrayed us as children and used us as sexual objects? Our failure to remember such abuse presented no problem. Surely the abuse was so shocking, so villainous, we could not believe it was happening. Hence, the theory held, we repressed all memory of the experience into the unconscious, where it would work its mischief over time, all unknown and even unsuspected.

If this wasn't Freudian in content, it was nonetheless Freudian in shape—not orthodox Freudianism, but what we might call "manneristic Freudianism." The mannerists lacked Freud's originality and literary gifts, of course, but they tried to follow him as best they could.

So, for instance, both the orthodox and the mannerists believed that Western society is the primary source of mental distress: Freud taught that society restricted the expression of our drives, producing conflicts and neurosis; the mannerists claimed that society protected the sexual predators by its paternalistic structure. Meanwhile, both believed in a dynamic unconscious roiling with suppressed secrets: Freud supposed that the unconscious hid our selfish impulses and hungers from consciousness and thus from censure by a repressive culture; the mannerists held that the unconscious hid the shocking memories from consciousness so that family life could go on. Finally, both believed that therapy should bring the unconscious issues to light: Freud said this would spare subjects from wasting psychic energy repressing their drives and so allow them to flourish in "love and work"; the mannerists believed that acknowledging the "repressed" abuse would lead to a life free of the nightmares, failures in personal relationships, and self-destructive behaviors generated by the unconscious memories.

The manneristic Freudians made intellectual moves defined by orthodox Freudianism, even while they rejected such politically incorrect Freudian ideas as penis envy. And so the memory wars were launched by the aggressive proposals of the manneristic Freudians. The signal event in this offensive against reason and plausibility was the publication in 1984 of Jeffrey Masson's book *The Assault on Truth: Freud's Suppression of the Seduction Theory.* As the archivist of the Freud papers (many of which are still secret), Masson was an insider among the orthodox Freudians, but he turned on his master's memory to resurrect Freud's original claim of childhood sexual abuse as the cause of neurosis. Indeed, Masson claimed that Freud *knew* it to be true but lacked the courage to press on with it. With the publication of this book—and the consequent dismissal of Masson as Freud's archivist—manneristic Freudianism and the concept of repressed memory moved to the front of psychiatry.

This first phase of the memory wars demonstrated how quickly an idea about mental life can grow and spread in the public, particularly if it offers an opportunity to identify new victims and new villains. The manneristic Freudians encountered few obstructions as their ideas gained support through the 1980s and early 1990s from psychiatrists and psychologists working in psychotherapy.

Many books were written to encourage the practice of recovering lost memories, the most successful of which—indeed, a continuing best-seller—was *The Courage to Heal: A Guide for Women Survivors of Child Sexual Abuse*, published in 1988 by two radical feminists with no qualifications in psychology and psychiatry. By 1991 some manneristic Freudians were claiming that up to half of the patients in psychiatric care were suffering from the effects of repressed or dissociated memories of sexual abuse.

It was in the late 1980s and early 1990s as well that many psychiatrists in teaching positions began to receive calls from families reporting how their adult offspring—mostly daughters—were accusing them of the most ferocious forms of sexual abuse when they were children. Casualties began to mount rapidly: mostly family breakup and estrangement but also growing mental derangement in the accusers. They were under pressure first to "remember" the details of the purported abuse they had "repressed" and then to "relive" these experiences in their psychotherapy sessions for cathartic relief. Why was it a surprise when patients treated in this fashion got worse, not better? More symptoms of depression colored with anger, resentment, and fear emerged, and suicide attempts began to occur. Long hospitalizations were often required. All these unfortunate outcomes replicated Freud's original experience with recovered-memory treatment a hundred years before.

The second phase of the memory wars was the organization of opposition to these ideas and practices. In 1992 a group of accused parents and concerned psychologists and psychiatrists founded the False Memory Syndrome Foundation (of which I am a board member) to "provide support and advice to accused family members and to disseminate scientific information about trauma and memory to the public at large." The argument of the foundation was that therapeutic techniques attempting to recover repressed memories actually led to the creation of psychologically compelling but false memories of childhood sex abuse, with all the destructive effects such false beliefs bring to the patient and the family.

The hope in this phase of the memory wars was that common sense would soon prevail and this misdirection of psychiatry from standard practices of evaluation and therapy would promptly stop. But the opposition to the idea of repressed memory received little or no support from official psychiatry or from the editorial policies of such professional journals as the *American Journal of Psychiatry*. Still, among the most useful efforts in the second phase of the memory wars was the publication of books about the misdirections of thought and misconstrual of evidence represented in the repressed memory claims. An outstanding contribution was Frederick Crews's series of articles in the *New York Review of Books*, ultimately brought together in 1995 as a book entitled *The Memory Wars: Freud's Legacy in Dispute.*

Also in this second phase, many patients treated for repressed memories came to realize that they had been misled by their therapists and retracted their claims against their fathers and mothers. Some of the most egregious examples garnered public attention, and their stories about how they came to have false memories under psychotherapeutic suggestions got attention in periodicals as diverse as *Esquire* and the *American Scholar.* Cumulatively, these attacks on repressed-memory syndrome began to take effect, and as the existence of false memories became obvious, the courts began to protect accused parents from prosecution by offspring. Later, many former patients launched civil lawsuits for malpractice against their hospitals and therapists, and juries gave them huge financial settlements.

Perhaps the greatest scandal of the memory wars lies in this: the official avenues of clinical and scientific debate failed to play a role in ending these practices, while public rebuke and punishment did. Enormous damage is done to a medical discipline when it is forced to advance and retreat under the gun of the malpractice courts—but when the psychiatric establishment was at best absent, and at worst complicit, in the widespread practice of a psychiatric abuse, what alternative was there?

The result was at least partially effective. No one these days is bragging about how skilled they are at bringing forth forgotten memories, and some of the crazier ideas, such as "multiple personality disorder" and "satanic ritual abuse," do not get much exposure anymore. But many practitioners still believe in the concept of repression (often translating it into another term, *dissociation*) and claim that all the obvious troubles that came to light and led to court action were due not to erroneous ideas but to incompetent practitioners. To this day, one meets intelligent people ready to accept repressed memories as common and to assume that the evidence for their regular occurrence with sexual trauma is strong. The scientists and practitioners who tried to show how these ideas about memory are wrong are still routinely slandered as "extremists," "biased," or "against children."

The courts, in other words, could only repress some of the worst practices of the repressed-memory diagnosis. The horrendous idea itself needed something more to destroy it—which is the cause of what we might call the third phase of the memory wars.

This phase began with closer study of the cases in the literature that purport to prove the existence of "repressed memories." The first key event of the third phase was the 1997 testimony of the distinguished psychiatrist Herbert Spiegel, which indicated that the classic case of "Sybil" (which purported to demonstrate repressed memories and multiple personalities) was contrived—almost fraudulently so—to gain publicity. Again and again, the standard cases of repressed memory dissolved under close study. Some of the afflicted patients were children caught up in a divorce and persuaded by one of the parents to accuse the other. Others proved ready to retract their accusations when they learned of alternative explanations for their troubles.

This aspect of the memory wars has occasionally turned nasty as the protagonists for "recovered memories" pressured university committees—claiming invasion of privacy when the published cases were assessed anew—to stop the investigators from exploring their claims. Nonetheless, one by one, all the central examples of repressed memories proved unsubstantial.

In *Remembering Trauma*, Richard McNally monitors this final phase of the memory wars. McNally is both an experienced clinician and a prominent scientific investigator of memory. He provides a comprehensive description of both normal memory and memory influenced by time, prejudicial influence, trauma, and emotions. He systematically reviews all the claims and the theories brought forth to defend repressed-memory therapy, and he shows just how distorted the thinking of its champions is. The result is a damning judgment against the basic concepts of the manneristic Freudians.

McNally is so thorough in his reviews of scientific knowledge about memory and every one of the claims for support of the repressed-memory idea—from clinical anecdotes to such neurobiological ideas as brain scars in the hippocampus—that a casual reader may weary. But veterans of the memory wars will be grateful to him for this thoroughness because he leaves no defense of repressed memory unassailed and thus brings fully to light what went wrong in psychiatry with the manneristic Freudians.

After reading McNally, one has a clear idea of the direction psychiatry must take. Psychiatrists need to cease seeking a generic explanation for mental disorder. They must align themselves instead with psychologists and neuropsychologists to explore the individual faculties of normal mental life—from perception and language, to emotion and drive, all the way down to memory. Most of all, psychiatry must become a *medicine*, moving toward a structure of reasoning and practice where knowledge of normal function leads to an understanding of just what has gone wrong in particular diseases. Richard McNally's *Remembering Trauma* is more than the final nail in the coffin of the repressed-memory craze. It is the blueprint for how psychiatry can best progress in the years to come.

The Weekly Standard, 2003

Dissociative Identity Disorder Is a Socially Constructed Artifact

Multiple personality disorder (MPD) (or, as DSM-IV will have it, dissociative identity disorder [DID]) has been the star diagnosis of the past decade. Many psychiatrists, who knew it as a rare but occasional presentation of a suggestible patient and had long agreed with the Mayer-Gross, Slater, and Roth textbook that multiple personalities "are artificial productions, the product of the medical attention that they arouse" (Mayer-Gross, Slater, & Roth, 1969), were surprised when case examples became so numerous that in some centers entire wards could be devoted to them. These psychiatrists soon learned that a belief held by psychotherapists that these patients had suffered repeated sexual abuse as children at the hands of trusted guardians was generating the enthusiasm for this diagnosis—an enthusiasm that bordered on a crusade. DID, so the theory runs, represents the incapacity of the patient to remember and acknowledge this frightful, abusive experience. The treatment—again following the assumed explanation—consists of reintegrating the mental life of the patient by drawing all the repressed experiences back into awareness and finding more effective ways of dealing with their implications than "dissociating" into alternative personalities.

I believe that the emergence of this entity into prominence and particularly the acceptance of this dubious explanation with little more than anecdotal evidence is another culturally driven misdirection of psychiatry and psychotherapy. It began as an idea held by just a few. Subsequently this idea spread widely among susceptible therapists who are ever hungry for fresh concepts that carry with them the sense of "I know a secret" and who were supported, even directed, to search for victims of abuse by sociopolitical movements identifying mediating institutions such as the family as exploitative and paternalistic. Now, as the harmful implications of the idea have come to be appreciated by psychiatrists and psychologists, even its champions are wavering in their enthusiasm, shifting their definitions of the condition as the force of counterarguments is felt and their reputations are threatened. As they shift, they often claim that they were misunderstood, that their work has been applied by "poor therapists" who lack their skills, or that critics need to understand just how subtle the actual concepts of multiplicity and personality are.

DID will eventually return to its prior status as an occasional oddity. How it came to have its moment of fame (and how it revealed a methodological Achilles' heel in the "operational criteria" approach of DSM-III and -IV) will, however, remain a subject of interest.

One can start by parsing the claim in the Mayer-Gross, Slater, and Roth text. It offered the standard formulation of DID (MPD) prior to the contributions of Cornelia Wilbur (Ludwig et al., 1972), Richard Kluft (1991), Frank Putnam (1989), David Spiegel (1991), and others. In this text, the authors claim that MPD is one of the many medical artifacts that psychiatrists are familiar with and occasionally inadvertently promote, that is, behaviors of patients in which symptoms of some natural illness are imitated. Other examples of artifacts include the hysterical "conversion" disorders, Briquet syndrome, factitious disorders, malingering, and so on.

All medical and psychiatric artifacts are behavioral efforts—conscious or unconscious—on the part of patients to capture medical or psychiatric attention and achieve the advantages offered by the "sick role" (Slavney, 1990). Common elements include vulnerabilities of temperament (particularly enhanced suggestibility and hypnotizability), mental distress in the form of anxiety or depression, and, most critically, access to cultural "idioms" suitable for depicting a person in distress and in need of help, protection, and solicitude.

Artifacts present either as complaints of a physical kind (pain, weakness, fainting, etc.) that compel medical diagnostic attention or as psychological manifestations (trances, fugues, alternative personalities, etc.) that attract psychiatric interest. The artifact serves to depict the patient as a victim either of a mysterious illness that "stumps the experts" or of such misadventures in life that the patient is entitled to assistance and sympathy. Mystery illnesses can include subtle but presumed endocrine or infectious disorders; misadventures can include agents of malevolence—ranging from uncaring parents to witches or extraterrestrials. The existence of the symptoms "proves" that "something is wrong" and often serves the interpersonal defenses of the patient by portraying many others (e.g., family members, nurses, physicians) as ignorant and uncaring, especially if they cast any doubt on the cause of the condition.

Patients with artifactual conditions always provoke apprehension among physicians, primarily because doctors fear overlooking a natural condition that is manifesting in an unusual way. But concerns also emerge because these patients, when hospitalized, tend to split the staff over issues of diagnosis and management and consume resources interminably.

However, rational management emerges once an artifact is identified and understood. Artifacts, it is known, serve to distract a patient from his or her actual problems. They may accomplish this by simply screening complicated affairs or by representing them in some partial, symbolic, or otherwise distorted form. The patients—vulnerable by temperament to suggestion and fantasy—are distressed, confused, and at odds with themselves. An artifactual construction, expressed in the form of either physical or psychological symptoms, provides a temporary resolution for their psychological condition and brings attention and support from physicians.

Medical and psychiatric attention, however, once turned away from the features of the artifact and toward the patient's actual difficulties—sometimes related to contemporary adjustment problems, sometimes to long-standing interpersonal conflicts—helps the patient to abandon the artifactual symptoms without any confrontation over them and to participate in effective psychotherapy. Hypnosis or Amytal are not used to seek more symptoms but can be employed to release the patient from a commitment to artifactual behaviors that preoccupy attention and interfere with therapy. Ultimately, after progress has been made on the issues that were overshadowed by the artifactual symptoms, these symptoms can be gently confronted and given meaning in relation to the understanding that has emerged in psychotherapy.

This is exactly how the occasional examples of DID seen prior to the contemporary rage for this diagnosis were treated. One did not hypnotize the patient to bring forth more "alters" or to "discover" traumas. One never talked to or in any other way worked with "alters," never charted their comments in separate files, called them by name, or accommodated their demands. This was considered as potentially indulging and sustaining the artifactual behavior, just as if one prescribed Dilantin for patients with pseudoseizures, hearing aids for patients with artifactual deafness, or crutches for the artifactually paralyzed. All efforts were exerted to review the present life of the patient and bring those issues to the forefront of therapeutic efforts. One expected and usually came to realize that personality disorders and conflicts of considerable complexity lay at the root of the presenting complaints. Despite some difficulties—often related to the patient's attempts to hold on to the artifactual condition or replace it with another—such treatments worked well.

This prescription for DID, however, is not followed on most "dissociative units" today. There, all is more complicated, controversial, and ambiguous but, it must be said, fundamentally oversimplified. The patients are viewed by everyone as most intriguing individuals. Much clinical attention—including hypnosis—is directed toward eliciting more and more "alters," seeking the ones that confirm these patients as victims of one of humanity's most vile crimes. Rounds can be taken up with much ritual such as finger wigwags ("ideomotor signaling") to "access" certain hidden "alters" without requiring their "full emergence." Much chaotic behavior on the part of the patient is either tolerated or heavily medicated, as it is thought to represent "alters" in action. These "alters" can be animals; thus, barking, howling, and roaring are acceptable behaviors among these patients. The vague term *dissociation* covers everything.

Despite all this activity, the patients and their records are not scrutinized for conflicts embedded within the hopes and wishes of their lives because DID is assumed to be the linear consequence of child abuse. Confirming evidence of the abuse—through critically evaluated external informants—is not sought because theory provides confidence. Finally, the treatment proposed is extensive, prolonged, expensive, and stuffed with drama—indeed, melodrama. It is all a huge mistake.

Start with dissociation. Ever since Janet, the concept of dissociation has been problematic. The major difficulty has always been what to include and what to exclude in the concept of dissociation. Because its assumptions are subtly tied to those of associationism, the concept of dissociation has been applied to almost every psychopathological symptom at one time or another. After all, one can always claim that some disruption of the "associative links" must lie behind any mental phenomena, even hallucinations and delusions, in which perceptions and reality fail to connect. Dissociation has, from its inception, been a concept in need of restraint.

In addition, many symptoms that are related to consciousness should be differentiated from dissociation and often are not. One such symptom is depersonalization/derealization. Depersonalization is a symptom—an affectively distressful sense of change in the awareness of the self and the environment such that they seem unreal. It occurs in a number of circumstances (Ackner, 1954): as an epileptic symptom, a drug-induced state, a complication of sleep deprivation, and so on. The "numbing" phenomena seen with acute grief and during and after a catastrophe or other trauma are expressions of depersonalization but are time-limited.

Dissociation is not depersonalization and vice versa. Dissociation is a concept and not a symptom. It attempts to explain how the usually "associated" parts of consciousness can become separated. Dissociation no more encompasses depersonalization—a qualitative alteration in the "sense of consciousness" itself—than it does other symptoms of consciousness such as faintness.

The phenomena to which Janet applied his first iterations of the explanatory concept "dissociation" included artifactual—then termed "hysterical"—paralyses and sensory losses as well as mental artifacts such as amnesias, fugue states, and misperceptions. In the United States, with the emergence of the concept of conversion as the purported explanation for motor and sensory artifacts, the term *dissociation* as in dissociative hysteria came to be restricted to mental artifacts. However, both conversion and dissociation are problematic terms that add confusion to our understanding of artifactual medical and psychiatric conditions.

This confusion is obvious with dissociation—a descriptive metaphor that can easily masquerade as an explanation. Thus, when a patient presents with "alters" as part of DID, these are "explained" as dissociative phenomena and the patient is said to have a dissociative disorder. However, the action of dissociation is identified by pointing to the "alters"—the very phenomena that the proposal of dissociation was to explain. One goes round and round this way: that which needs to be explained is given a hypothetical mechanism, the only expression of which is the symptom that provoked the search for an explanation originally. The concept of dissociation lacks methodological and conceptual specificity (Jaspers, 1963). This makes it a perfect ingredient for artifacts. It provides patients and therapists with a compelling "idiom" but does not survive careful scrutiny.

Most of the heat in the DID controversy, however, rests on the issue of hidden child abuse—abuse pushed out of consciousness by dissociation and repression. The problem here is that the abuse is very often presumed and not confirmed. Simply put, these patients are not "worked up" in a clinically standard way through the use of differential diagnoses, external informants, and alternative therapeutic planning. Why this is so often turns on several factors in the therapeutic culture at the moment, including views about maintaining a therapeutic alliance by "believing the patient" and assumptions about repression, dissociation, and the memory of trauma. Yet there are no compelling data available from which one could confidently say that experiences of sexual abuse are commonly forgotten or that this abuse or any other trauma regularly provokes DID. Anecdotes abound, as in the provocative story of Sybil (Schreiber, 1973), but these hardly suffice, particularly when full evaluations of the patients including external informants have not been attempted.

Linda Meyer Williams's work (1994) often mentioned as demonstrating the frequency with which sexual abuse is forgotten, cannot be considered anything more than a pilot study because no other injured children were followed as controls along with the sexually abused patients and because the number of failures to report the abuse did not exceed those found in other studies following up on patients with previous accidents or hospitalizations. That individuals can forget all kinds of misfortunes has never been denied. In fact, this had been considered an advantage to such individuals in contrast to those with recurring memories of their traumas. For all these reasons, Williams's work cannot be used to prove that sexual trauma is unique either in being frequently repressed or in provoking particular mental disorders. For example, none of her subjects complained of DID.

In truth, the idea that trauma explains many psychological problems has been considered a gross oversimplification almost from the start of modern psychotherapy. Such a concept glossed over the complicated aspects of conflicted people and was rightfully condemned by Freud and others in the face of accumulated experience. Obviously childhood traumas, whether physical or sexual, can have bad implications for later life. No one is denying or has denied this. But let there be no mistake: imagined childhood sexual abuse can be equally disruptive to mental life. In fact, a "feeling" of abuse without a memory accesses another contemporary cultural idiom—we are all victims, whether we know it or not—that will bolster an appeal for support, one that is difficult to criticize without being regarded by many as unsympathetic and by some as ignorant, vicious, or criminal. Such an appeal, for all its obvious manipulative characteristics, is hard to resist and explains both the fervor of its champions and the caution of its adversaries.

Finally, the treatments of DID, especially within so-called dissociative units, are often interminable—months and even years of inpatient care—just what one might expect when artifacts, rather than natural psychological conditions, are the focus of the program. We await controlled studies that test the idea that DID should be given special treatments different from those long recognized to be effective with artifacts and standard in the profession. Many therapists, in fact, can already attest that paying attention to the current adjustment disorders, the particular personal vulnerabilities, and the abiding conflicts and compromises of the patients rather than to the elaboration of "alters"—out to and including animal alters who bark and meow—can lead to recovery (Ganaway, 1994).

Psychiatry has once again indulged a therapeutic craze. Proponents of a new idea and a new treatment—always a temptation for psychotherapists, since the proper treatment of psychic conflict is difficult—have provoked a huge controversy and yet do not consider or adequately confront the evidence that they have promoted and sustained a psychiatric artifact in vulnerable people (Kenny, 1986). They have burdened patients and families by providing misguided therapy with hurtful implications. They have distracted attention from the reality of child abuse by overdiagnosing it and seldom attempting to confirm it. As patients and families eventually emerge from the injuries produced by this misdirected oversimplification of psychiatry, there will be much to repair and much to acknowledge in order to restore the integrity and good reputation of psychotherapy.

Journal of Practical Psychiatry and Behavioral Health, 1995

REFERENCES

Ackner, B. (1954). Depersonalization. *Journal of Mental Science* 100:838–872.

Ganaway, G. K. (1994). Transference and countertransference shaping influences on dissociative syndromes. In *Dissociation: Clinical and theoretical perspectives*, ed. S. Lynn and J. Rhue, 317–337. New York: Guilford.

Hart, B. (1959). *The psychology of insanity*. Cambridge: Cambridge University Press.

Jaspers, K. (1963). *General psychopathology*. Chicago: University of Chicago Press.

Kenny, M. G. (1986). *The passion of Ansel Bourne*. Washington, D.C.: Smithsonian Institution Press.

Kluft, R. P. (1991). Multiple personality disorder. In *American Psychiatric Press review of psychiatry*, ed. A. Tasman and S. Goldfinger, 10:161–188. Washington, D.C.: American Psychiatric Press.

Ludwig, A. M., J. M. Brandsma, C. B. Wilbur, F. Bendfeldt, and D. H. Jameson. (1972). The objective study of a multiple personality. *Archives of General Psychiatry* 26:298–310.

Mayer-Gross, W., E. Slater, and M. Roth. (1969). *Clinical psychiatry*. 3rd ed. London: Bailliere, Tindall and Cassell.

Putnam, F. W. (1989). *Diagnosis and treatment of multiple personality disorder*. New York: Guilford.

Schreiber, F. R. (1973). *Sybil*. Chicago: Henry Regnery.

Slavney, P. R. (1990). *Perspectives on hysteria*. Baltimore: Johns Hopkins University Press.

Spiegel, D. (1991). Dissociation and trauma. In *American Psychiatric Press review of psychiatry*, ed. A. Tasman and S. Goldfinger, 10:261–275. Washington, D.C.: American Psychiatric Press.

Williams, L. M. (1994). Recall of childhood trauma: A prospective study of women's memories of child sexual abuse. *Journal of Consulting and Clinical Psychology* 62:1167–1176.

Part IV

PATHFINDERS AND PATHWAYS

I long ago concluded that the triumph of various misdirections in psychiatry should be in part blamed on the surrender of general medicine to psychiatric authority. Especially in academic medicine, where one might expect the standards to be highest and the resistance to the market of excessive promises greatest, leaders did not demand anything like the standards of proof that they demanded of internists, surgeons, pediatricians, and the like. The lucidity of scientific thought that directed all decisions in the rest of medicine was often abandoned when psychiatric matters were discussed—hence the strange cultic forms that evolved, finding support in the citadels of American academic medicine.

It's not as though there were not other examples and useful admonitions against these trends in psychiatry which could have been considered when decisions of how to teach and investigate it were being made. In this part of the book I discuss the contributions to thought provided by a leading psychiatrist, Karl Jaspers, and a leading internist, William Osler. Much of what they were saying was ignored for many decades within the twentieth century by psychiatrists and others worried that the "medical model" would not work in the psychiatric clinic. Much that has happened in the last quarter of the century and during my tenure at Johns Hopkins has ended that issue.

But still psychiatry remains very different from medicine in thought and practice. These differences, I believe, still rest on misunderstanding of the conditions psychiatrists treat. Ultimately the ever critical foundational question for all doctors is: Just what kind of disorder is the proffered therapy aiming to correct? The failure to demand that psychiatrists address this question is the source of most of the present difficulties. The classificatory manual for the discipline—the Diagnostic and Statistical Manual of Mental Disorders *(DSM)—turns out to be a kind of field guide useful at the moment for correcting the fissiparous tendencies in psychiatric discourse, but it is very different from the classification methods in medicine and thus unable to answer the fundamental question posed above in any substantive way.*

The essays to follow offer the sources of our current thought and ultimately the way that we have come to teach psychiatry at Johns Hopkins.

Genius in a Time, Place, and Person

Foreword to Karl Jaspers's *General Psychopathology*, Volume 1

For those who would understand psychiatry, this book is indispensable. Although it draws from the clinical thought and practices of the late nineteenth and early twentieth centuries, its delineation of the methods for comprehending mental disorders remains unmatched to this day. It is, in fact, a product of a special time, place, and person.

The Time

Consider first its time. The year *General Psychopathology* was published—1913—was pivotal in the history of psychiatry. It was the culmination of the most productive decade of this century. It was also the last year before the great German tradition of university-based empirical psychiatry was drowned by the chaos of war, economic depression, Nazi barbarism, and the Cold War's division of East and West Germany.

In the ten years from 1903 to 1913, the investment of fifty years of preparation and prior work bore fruit. In that decade, Emil Kraepelin published the eighth and definitive edition of his textbook *Psychiatrie: Ein Lehrbuch für Studirende und Ärtze* (1909), Eugen Bleuler introduced the term *schizophrenia* (1906), and Alois Alzheimer described the condition that now bears his name (1907). These outstanding contributions to empirical psychiatry, though, were matched in the same decade by a maturing interpretive psychiatry. Sigmund Freud's fledgling movement, "psychoanalysis," gained international reputation through its spread among neurologists, private practitioners, and the sophisticated middle classes of Europe, through the interest of American physicians and society prompted by Freud's 1909 visit to Clark University, and through the revisionism and generation of alternative ideas provided by the breakaway in this decade of former students of Freud—Alfred Adler and Carl Gustav Jung. Freud, Jung, and Adler did more than propose explanations for psychiatric disorder; they generated a movement of thought about human mental life, well enough advanced by 1913 for any perspicacious student to predict its eventual power and claims.

As is obvious from this mere sketch, the initial collision between empirical and interpretive psychiatry occurred in this decade and originated in two linear Teutonic thinkers (Kraepelin and Freud). Their contention demanded resolution, but—with the exception of this great book—no such effort was made, in part because of the social chaos that enveloped the original champions and their followers. Enervating as it is to teaching and practice, this psychiatric conflict festers to the present day, with empirical and interpretive psychiatry retitled "biologic" and "dynamic." The monolithic tyrannies of the originators persist.

The Place

If 1913 was a propitious year for someone to identify and resolve the warring concepts of psychiatry, then the place where this book was written was itself ideal. The Psychiatric Clinic of the University of Heidelberg, the preeminent German university and academic center, was under the direction of Franz Nissl, he of the Nissl stain in neurohistology. Nissl was an intense, hardworking, odd character who started on the wrong side in the battle of the neuron theory and learned from his mistakes. He was the perfect chief for such a clinical research institution: a methodical scientist himself who had learned about the difficulties of discovery.

A man of integrity without envy, Nissl could get others to join him in the enterprise of clinical and investigative psychiatry. He emphasized his colleagues' strengths rather than harping on their weaknesses. With these traits, combined with a passionate interest in scientific effort and achievement, he created an atmosphere of vigorous and free discussion among his faculty. For all that his own creativity was modest, his choices of colleagues, his enthusiasm for new enterprises, and his lack of autocratic tyrannies helped to create an environment in which inventiveness of all kinds flourished.

Nissl was not initially enthusiastic about this work of Karl Jaspers, wondering whether it was merely philosophical hairsplitting or "monkey business," as he called abstract treatises. Once he had read it, however (carrying the galley sheets around in the pocket of his white coat for weeks), he became its champion. Jaspers noted that Franz Nissl in Heidelberg in 1913 was just the right leader to produce a "genius of place."

The Person

The time and place inspired a special person to write this book. Karl Jaspers came to Heidelberg right from medical school in 1908. He brought with him a unique set of qualities. Although initially interested in philosophy, he had turned to study medicine, which, he believed, best illuminated life itself and the challenges of human existence. However, he was chronically ill with bronchiectasis and could not assume heavy clinical duties. Jaspers won Nissl's begrudging permission to work in the library rather than the clinic or laboratory. His skills as an open-minded, critical, indeed often skeptical, thinker about psychiatric opinions and practices came to the fore. Jaspers soon realized, and as promptly said, that the library volumes (and the psychiatric periodical literature) were filled with "unfounded chatter." This "chatter" derived from the mushrooming of independent self-referential schools of thought about patients— each with its own terminology. Jaspers discerned that there was no commonly accepted, science-based, logical approach to psychiatry, not even a common observational method for identifying the manifestations of psychiatric disorders.

The problem was not just in the library. In the clinics as well, psychiatrists on one day seemed to work according to a Kraepelinian diagnostic formula but on the next proposed some theoretical explanation that took nothing from the previous day's ideas. It seemed to Jaspers that psychiatrists struggled to make sense of their discipline. They were aware of concepts and facts but were unsure of when particular explanations for disorder might apply, and they adopted treatments and research programs almost on impulse. Coincidentally Jaspers also appreciated why many of his more gifted contemporaries restricted their work to brain studies. At least they could get their hands around the brain, even if the problem of importance to the patient lay somewhere else.

"To make real progress psychiatrists must learn to think," he said during one discussion with colleagues. "Jaspers ought to be spanked," replied his contemporaries.

Jaspers sensed that psychiatry inhabited a middle ground between science, where laws of nature are discerned, and history, where fateful events are conceived as emerging from human choices and actions. That is, Jaspers knew that some mental disorders derive from brain diseases and therefore psychiatrists should be close allies with neurologists. But he also knew that mental distress could emerge as consequences of some conflict between an individual's wishes and actual life circumstances, so psychiatrists should naturally share interests with students in the social and cultural disciplines. In fact, Jaspers saw more coherence and conceptual development among neurologists and social scientists than among most psychiatrists. The students in the disciplines surrounding psychiatry tended to reflect on the methods behind their opinions and thus learned to judge them.

Jaspers turned to three prominent social scientists to organize his thought: the philosopher Edmund Husserl, the historian Wilhelm Dilthey, and the political scientist Max Weber. Husserl comes first because Jaspers took from him an approach to examining patients. Husserl taught that the contents of the conscious mind of others could be accessed and described by what he called at first "descriptive psychology" and later "phenomenology." Jaspers followed Husserl's lead and, with modifications for the clinical setting, defined a phenomenological approach to interviewing and examining psychiatric patients.

The phenomenological method hinges on the human capacity for self-expression—a means of communicating one's experiences to another. This capacity makes it possible for patients to describe the contents of their minds and for psychiatrists listening to these descriptions to enter the mental life of such patients. Through this process psychiatrists can emphatically penetrate (almost coexperience) their patients' thoughts, perceptions, and feelings and note the similarities and differences among the "phenomena" they find.

The phenomenologically inspired interaction between psychiatrists and patients calls for efforts that go beyond the definition and cataloging of disordered mental events such as delusions and hallucinations. The psychiatrist attempts to grasp these events as experiences within the consciousness of the patient—a kind of "living with" the events as the patient recounts them.

Jaspers, following Husserl, proposed that psychiatrists could achieve such an understanding of their patients' mental life if they approached the task of inquiry without prejudice of theory but rather by attempting to gain from a patient a full description of his or her mental experience. The process is not some secret seeking but rather a true "meeting of minds." In this book Jaspers lays out a treasury of characteristic disruptive experiences within human consciousness accessible to psychiatrists prepared to take up such a "walk in your shoes" stance with their patients.

Once he clarified the "phenomenological" approach and described the characteristic features of disordered thoughts, perceptions, and emotions, Jaspers's next issue was to differentiate the several prevailing explanations for mental disorders. Again he had little help from the psychiatric literature, where he found a muddle of conflicting schools of thought. Here he turned to Dilthey and Weber. These social scientists taught that drawing explanatory "connections" between events—for example, concluding that the loss of a parent in childhood produced a revengeful character in the adult—was a hazardous business if not done methodically and systematically.

The social scientists had two methods at hand. An empirical, statistical demonstration of the regular co-occurrences of certain events in a population might provide evidence for the "connection" between them, but an empathic assertion that a particular experience had special meaning in the life story of an individual might suggest even more powerfully the link between an experience and a later behavior. Jaspers's goal became the appropriation and practical differentiation of these two social science methods of explanation so as to make them available to psychiatric teaching, investigation, and practice.

Thus, he could support Kraepelin's opinions on heredity and mental illness based on the statistical study of hundreds of patients and their families. And, as well, he could identify what Freud and Adler were claiming for "connections" between early life experience and the development of a disorder such as hysteria or anxiety. Jaspers, taking the terminology from Dilthey, distinguished these two modes of work by speaking of Kraepelin's method as "explanation" (*erklären*). "Explanation," Jaspers noted, was the attempt to discern nature's laws acting impersonally, through "causal connections," to produce a mental disorder.

Jaspers identified Freud's method as "understanding" (*verstehen*). "Understanding," Jaspers taught, grasped for "meaningful connections" in an attempt to demonstrate that disorder emerged because of a conflict between experience and a specific individual's hopes and desires—a conflict and its emotional consequences that could be empathically appreciated for the person even though not statistically demonstrable.

By differentiating "explanation" and "understanding," Jaspers emphasized that there was a critical epistemological divide within the field of psychiatry and that psychiatrists could bridge this divide only by appreciating these different methods at their disposal. But woe to the psychiatrist who confused "understanding" with "explanation" (as Jaspers believed Freud to have done) because then false claims and misdirected hypotheses would once again muddle this field.

Thus, from each method Jaspers identified contributions to psychiatry. But he emphasized those contributions as having limits implicit in the method itself. For example, he noted that Kraepelinian labels might slight the personal suffering of an individual, whereas Freudian interpretations might overlook a neurobiologic process.

Jaspers also emphasized those limits because he held that neither provided full views of human mental life and its potentials. He believed and emphasized in his phenomenological studies that the individual human being—even afflicted by mental disorder—was always more than we can know. In essence, Jaspers's object was to show psychiatrists exactly what they know, how they know it, and what they do not know and cannot claim. He wrote this book with these aims in mind.

Aftermath

General Psychopathology was a splendid achievement for anyone but amazing for a man of barely thirty years of age. A fascinating fact, though, is that it culminated the psychiatric productivity of its author, who, with the exception of revising the text (with some expansion) for subsequent editions (this is the seventh), left psychiatric work forever. He became a distinguished leader in twentieth-century existential philosophy. He was also a voice of reason in the catastrophic events that overcame his university and his country. He was a prodigy in many ways, but as a physician, who led a philosophical movement and denounced tyranny when others were silent, he was most special.

Jaspers always claimed that the work in *General Psychopathology* was his avenue to understanding human nature. An open, unblinkered view of mental illness gave him a comprehension of mental health. As well, his dedication to identifying limits to imperious claims about human beings protected him from the huge ideological errors of this century. His emphasis on the phenomena of human consciousness helped him grasp an essential characteristic of human mental life—its promise. His commitment to this promise provoked his enmity to the totalitarian systems that sprang up in the West (fascism, national socialism, Marxism-Leninism).

From the same allegiance to promise he also opposed physician-scientists who, emphasizing a fragmentary knowledge of human biology, slighted the value and grounds for hope in the lives of their patients. Thus, right from 1913, Jaspers attacked the growing power of the eugenics movement, which engaged psychiatrists around the world seeking "racial hygiene." His strong and persisting enmity toward racism in all its forms came from the same source and was based on his recognition of the fundamental unity of human mental experiences played out in individual lives and purposes.

His quarrels with psychoanalysis grew over time and increased with each edition of *General Psychopathology*. (They can also be reviewed in his philosophical works, such as *Man in the Modern Age* [1931].) The quarrel began in the first edition, in which he challenged the views of Freud and his followers that they had a scientific —that is, "causal" or "explanatory" rather than a "meaningful"— approach to mental disorders. Later, when the requirement for a training analysis became psychoanalytic policy, Jaspers attacked the movement both for its indoctrinating methods toward its students and for its fundamental nihilism (deriving even what is best in a person from base origins that only psychoanalysis can unveil).

At the very heart of all his teaching is Jaspers's radical commitment to two great themes, freedom and responsibility. These two themes must interrelate either for a person to reach his or her innate promise or for all of us to build a society worthy of mankind. The first of the two themes declares that the essence of human beings is freedom. Unlike all other creatures, men and women face an unpredictable future and have unlimited opportunities for progress. Jaspers's sense of human freedom aroused his hatred for simplistic notions about our nature and for coercive forces that would restrict our development to certain paths. He foresaw situations in which thinking about human beings as animals would eventually lead to treating them as such—culling them as if they were a flock or a herd.

The second theme—responsibility—reflects his appreciation that the way things are formed—families forged, societies built, cities sustained, and the future realized—depends in the last analysis on the decisions and deeds of individuals. "Each individual—by his way of life, his daily small deeds, by his great decisions, testifies to himself as to what is possible. By this, his present actuality, he contributes unknowingly toward the future." This idea—that there is no law of nature or law of history which determines what is and what will be but rather it is the many and repeated choices of free individuals which make or break this world—was fundamental to Jaspers's thought as a psychiatrist and as a philosopher. It made him inspect the choices suggested to and imposed on people by authorities of all kinds—scientific authorities as much as political authorities—and ultimately set him at odds with tyrannies, both the tyrannies of governments and the tyrannies of the crowd.

The central problem of modernity is how to tie freedom to self-government. In *General Psychopathology*, Jaspers addresses this issue as he describes the conceptual foundations of psychotherapy. He discloses that order in mental life is a consequence of enlightened freedom, not an imposition on it. Here Jaspers voices opinions that he derives from that quintessential modern source, psychotherapy, but which have had earlier advocates and other derivations (Thucydides from war, Augustine from the ruins of an imperial civilization, Jefferson from revolution). The main point of these advocates—and the essence of Jaspers's thought—is that people are free but can learn that they are responsible for the consequences of their actions.

These ideas, the promise in human nature and its realization through the interplay of freedom and responsibility, with all their implications for both psychiatric practice and a democratic society, are not found in the clinical writings of Jaspers's contemporaries

Kraepelin or Freud. This is another seldom noted, distinguishing feature of his work in both psychiatry and philosophy. Thus Jaspers alone advances the wisdom about patients needed to dispel the contemporary agitations around psychiatry that characteristically clamor for rights and disregard implications. These include the antipsychiatry of Michel Foucault and Thomas Szasz, the demand for physician-assisted suicide in the Netherlands, and the subtle forms of eugenics that the Human Genome Project has in store.

Conclusion

I call this book indispensable even though it was written eighty-four years ago—before the discovery of the EEG, DNA, or norepinephrine. I hold this view because, despite these many scientific advances, most of the problems that Jaspers noted in 1913 remain as problems to psychiatry today. We have more information than Jaspers found crowding the shelves in Heidelberg, but we still disagree about how best to order this information so as to encourage its steady progress and to read its fundamental messages.

Jaspers noted that psychiatrists must "develop and order knowledge guided by the methods through which it is gained—to learn the process of knowing and thereby to clarify the material." The twentieth century brought more facts to us. But a systematic appreciation of the methods of observation and interpretation that psychiatrists employ is essential to transform these facts into knowledge and its ultimate implications. No one since Jaspers has done it better.

REFERENCES

Jaspers, K. (1968). The phenomenological approach in psychopathology. *British Journal of Psychiatry* 114:1313–1323.
——. (1981). Philosophical autobiography. In *The philosophy of Karl Jaspers*, ed. Paul A. Schilpp. La Salle, Ill.: Open Court Publishing Co.
Shepherd, M. (1982a). Karl Jaspers: General psychopathology. *British Journal of Psychiatry* 141:310–312.
——. (1982b). The sciences and general psychopathology. In *Handbook of psychiatry*, vol. 1, ed. M. Shepherd and O. L. Zangwill. Cambridge: Cambridge University Press.

Slavney, P. R., and P. R. McHugh. (1987). Explanation and understanding. In *Psychiatric polarities*, 29–44. Baltimore: Johns Hopkins University Press.

Wiggins, O. P., and M. A. Schwartz. (1995). Chris Walker's interpretation of Karl Jaspers' phenomenology: A critique. *Philosophy, Psychiatry, and Psychology* 2:319–346.

———. (1997). Edmund Husserl's influence on Karl Jaspers' phenomenology. *Philosophy, Psychiatry, and Psychology* 4:15–36.

William Osler and the New Psychiatry

Of all the interactions of medicine with a subspecialty, those with psychiatry have been the most turbulent. Periods of separation and repudiation have been followed by periods of recommitment and rejoining. Such symbolic events as the separation of the National Institute of Mental Health from the National Institutes of Health, psychiatrists' rejection of identifying marks of the physician in the hospital, and the fortunately short-lived period when the internship requirement for psychiatrists was abandoned mark phases of repudiation. The development of psychiatric units on general hospitals, the growth of interest in psychosomatic disorders, and the enthusiastic commitment of time to psychiatric teaching within medical school curricula mark phases of recommitment.

Much of the turbulence in these periods comes from mutual fascination. There is a passionate energy in the phases of attraction and rejection that has given the association of medicine and psychiatry the flavor of romance more often than of kinship. For all that romance is exciting and allows one to enjoy the status of an intriguing, if occasionally capricious, companion, I want to emphasize the affinity and subdiscipline relationship of psychiatry to medicine by reviewing a time in medicine's past when issues similar to those shaping psychiatry's present were found.

I shall do this, though, not to muster the infuriating *tu quoque* retort that always exacerbates a quarrel between partners but to point out that psychiatry, as a subdiscipline of medicine, is following a course of development similar to that taken by medicine. This observation permits a prediction of a future for psychiatry that will transform our interactions with medicine from the unpredictable and wild shifts of adventure and enchantment to the more steady, constructive, and naturally fertile collaboration of kinship, with interdependence and harmony. It is perhaps about time.

To explain what I mean, we must look back into the late nineteenth century when William Osler was a vigorous and influential spokesman for a particular approach to medical education and practice that finally won the day in this country and abroad. The exact contributions of the Oslerians and like-minded contemporaries vary from place to place, but all of them depended upon a fundamental set of conceptions about medicine derived from a particular tradition linked to Sydenham, Harvey, and Linacre. These conceptions have not only succeeded but have become part of the fabric of our medical institutions; the revolutionary character they had in their time is often forgotten now. Therefore, the sense that psychiatry is moving in a direction similar to medicine may not be appreciated.

William Osler and His Ideas

Osler was interested in psychiatric matters. He was one of the early writers on Huntington disease, often spoke of the personality and characteristic emotional responses of people prone to angina and coronary thrombosis, and made a key clinical point that people express common disorders in unique ways depending on their personality, life habits, and experiences. Thus, he was ready to note and teach the difference between pathogenic and pathoplastic features in all kinds of diseases. But the psychiatric aspects of Osler's teaching are minor themes in his intellectual contributions to medicine.

Other interesting, identifying, but still incidental contributions of Osler can be noted by the student of medical history. He is remembered as a physician who brought teaching back to the bedside, reemphasizing the essential practical side of medical teaching. His textbook *The Principles and Practice of Medicine* (1892) may be cited as a compendium of then up-to-date information, remarkable for being composed by one person rather than the committees now required. He is sometimes seen as a person who lectured on the proper behavior of physicians, emphasizing Victorian, Kiplingesque attitudes with such ideals as the need to work and a commitment to equanimity. Some are repelled because many of Osler's essays to students are a touch lofty and righteous, calling for virtues in others that he had by nature. However, these things, if overemphasized, obscure his fundamental contribution as well as his cheerful disposition. Osler was not simply an encyclopedic and careful observer of clinical conditions or a high-minded scout master. He modeled a particular challenge to the medical education of the times and pointed out the ways and means to meet this challenge which we all have since followed, to the great advantage of the discipline.

Osler defined the problem of medical education of his day primarily as an excessive emphasis on therapeutics in both the training and many of the actions of physicians. He thought the emphasis on treatment that had little proof of efficacy led to unfortunate consequences, namely, the growth of denominations within medicine. Members of denominations resisted the advance of medical knowledge because they were ideologically committed to particular therapeutic theories rather than active in testing them.

Osler referred to the nineteenth-century treatment programs, from the homeopaths to the bleeders to the proponents of fresh air and spa water to the various deliverers of salves and ointments, as "pop-gun pharmacists who sometimes hit the disease and often hit the patient" (Osler, 1895). All directed attention away from medicine's ignorance about the causes and mechanisms of disease and the need for research into these features in order to find the proper modes of treatment and prevention. He deplored the separate communities and the distinctions in the titles (eclectic, homeopathic, etc.) of physicians and hoped for a time when physicians would be unified by their background and commitment to a common educational and practicing tradition.

To bring about such a day, Osler proposed that there should be two major elements of a medical education and therefore two major intellectual faculties of all physicians. He saw the marrying of these two faculties in practice as fundamental to all physicians and as the means to advancement that would produce rational therapeutics and preventive medicine, among other things.

The first element of a medical education, and the one he could most enhance personally, was the teaching of the natural history of disease. He believed a physician must be skilled at identifying and describing characteristic presentations of diseases, at identifying sequences of symptoms each disease traverses, and at discerning within a particular disease those features that differentiate it from others.

In this respect, Osler was expressing the tradition of Thomas Sydenham. Osler's choice of bedside teaching, which facilitates observing and conferring in a way impossible in lectures, was a logical outcome of this idea. He knew that individual presentations of disease are a complex of the pathognomic features and the individual expressions, stating, "as no two faces, so no two cases are alike in all respects, and unfortunately it is not only the disease itself which is varied, but the subjects themselves have pecularities which modify its actions" (Osler, 1895). It was the reiteration of this idea that led Osler to take his students to the bedside to show them the individual presentations of common diseases until they could differentiate what was related to the disease proper and what was special to the particular patient.

The second element of a medical education was a knowledge of the basic sciences to illuminate disorders and help explain the genesis of their pathognomic signs and sequences, commonalities, and distinctions. Osler thought the medical student should be acquainted with chemistry, pathology, pathophysiology, and the emerging sciences of bacteriology, immunology, epidemiology, and genetics. He was a disciple of William Harvey with the view that knowledge of underlying issues is crucial to students of disease and can be acquired only by laboratory experience and field study, the "hands-on" opportunity to see how science and its techniques are linked to the development and correction of clinical opinion.

Both these ideas are now basic to medical education and to the intellectual characteristics of physicians. However, Osler was lucky in his time. He was proposing these concepts along with other thoughtful educators, such as his colleagues at Johns Hopkins and Charles Eliot at Harvard. More fundamentally, Virchow had enlivened pathology by moving its focus from a gross to a cellular basis, Koch had nailed down the principles of bacteriology, and, with the rediscovery of Mendelian genetics, that discipline was emerging from the twilight of myths. If Osler had been born a hundred years earlier, his message might not have been as fruitful. Also as chairman of medicine at the newly formed medical school at Johns Hopkins, one of a "happy band" of educational innovators (Fleming, 1987, pp. 96–118), and with his personal characteristics, he was one of the few who could lead a revolution in education and medical practice to replace medical denominations and their pretensions with a clear sense of our knowledge and ignorance. He pointed out the logical generative path to the discoveries of therapeutics and preventive medicine that is now almost commonplace.

The Success of Osler

One can note the success of the marriage of basic science and the natural history of disease in many different areas. A prime example is the recent success of clinical and basic science in elucidating the pathogenesis of acquired immunodeficiency syndrome (AIDS) within four years of its recognition as an epidemic. The virus is identified, its target cell is appreciated, and its pathologic mechanisms are understood in relation to the symptoms it manifests. All these findings rested on Oslerian directives that were conceptual and educational. The ultimate harvests show what can be accomplished by someone whose leadership is based on a grasp of the contemporary obstacles to progress and who has the personal characteristics to overcome them. Osler's directives turned out to be more important than any single experiment or clinical study he might have done.

Another achievement of the "new" medicine personified by Osler was to stop the medical fads and sects that proliferated in the nineteenth century and before. As long as medicine focused primarily on therapy that was symptomatic, untested, and theoretical and probably depended on placebo for any efficacy, then idiosyncratic views on health, illness, and cure were regular outcomes of the discouragement felt by the sick. In America, these included the peculiar doctrines of chiropractic and osteopathy as well as recurrent enthusiasms for new ways of living and believing thought to promote health, which had their most powerful exemplar in Mary Baker Eddy and Christian Science. This tendency to outrageous enthusiasms had to bow before the success of post-Oslerian medicine. New faddish theories now spring up only from the fringes and counterculture and gain little popular support. Such is the ultimate success of building rational therapeutics upon comprehensive biological medicine.

Before going on to draw some analogies to psychiatry, I want to mention another of Osler's characteristics that was crucial to his role in the transition phase of medicine. Osler valued and honored the practitioners of his period and of the past. He saw the new era emerging and pointed out the path medicine should and would follow, but never with anything but respect and affection for those trained previously. He would never hear ill of them. He was not an isolated academic but a doctor who knew the practice of his contemporaries and its worth. He therefore won their support. He honored the "old-fashioned" values tied to the doctor's role and responsibility to patients even as he helped create a new technologically sophisticated discipline (Ludmerer, 1985, p. 135). He was a genial and gentle midwife to an emerging era, providing new skills to physicians but never overlooking the manner and values for which those skills were to be employed.

Psychiatry's Pre-Oslerian Status

I hope now that it is possible to see how psychiatry may seem a pre-Oslerian discipline. Its practitioners, worthy and kindly disposed toward patients, remain divided by denominations resting on therapy. It is beset by partisans for distinct treatments and approaches to patients. Certainly one of the loudest of these partisans, if hardly the most coherent voice in American psychiatry, proclaims that mental illness is a "myth" and that psychiatrists, his colleagues, are in league with repressive forces of society to deprive people of civil rights. In the name of "liberty" and his counsel, we have abandoned thousands of impaired and mentally deranged people to their fate; they wander our cities clinging to a few tattered possessions.

Psychiatry is the only discipline in which one practitioner asks another "what is your philosophy" or "what is your orientation" shortly after being introduced. This question is unsettling, for it identifies psychiatry as a denominational discipline rather than an integrated group of practitioners identified by their common education within a specialty. No one asks a cardiologist or gastroenterologist what his or her philosophy is even though differences of opinion and choices of approach to a particular patient or problem enliven daily rounds.

This is not so in psychiatry. The question "what is your orientation" anticipates an answer such as "I am a biological psychiatrist" or "I am behaviorally oriented" or more often now "I am eclectic," with the realization that one's answer identifies one's overall point of view about mental life and psychiatric conditions, and particularly how one views the cause of mental disorder and treats patients. The centers in American psychiatry seize mantles of particular therapies and call themselves biological or psychodynamic, exuding a sense of exclusion to others which bewilders all onlookers whatever their interest in the discipline.

Yet psychological and pharmacological treatments remain quite symptomatic in kind; the most effective were discovered by accident. They often resemble the "pop-gun pharmacy" of Osler's time, sometimes hitting the disease, sometimes hitting the patient, and us never knowing which is which. From outside psychiatry, new faddish theories about mental disorder and strange and fanciful treatment suggestions emerge almost annually. They are usually tied to charismatic people who write lively anecdote-filled books relating their conversion to particular worldviews and attitudes and who resemble the founders of osteopathy, chiropractic, or Christian Science.

The Emergence of Oslerian Principles in Psychiatry

I certainly do not wish to paint too bleak a picture of or provoke contempt for current psychiatry. It has had some wonderful achievements, including the continuing and traditional commitment to the care of the impaired and the recent emphasis on operational diagnosis and differentiation of disorders that approaches Osler's first principle. Also, I want to note some of the basic science advances. First, the differentiation of the neural systems in the brain that carry distinct neurochemical transmitters and thus may act as the site for both specific pathology in disease and for pharmacological treatment. Second, the appearance of new technologies, such as positron emission tomography, that illuminate the dynamic interactions of transmitter substances and receptors. Third, the growing interaction of psychiatry with neurology seen in the studies of Alzheimer disease, depression in Parkinson disease, and the manifestations and mechanisms of delirium. Fourth, the new information in genetics that emphasizes subtleties long known to internists is now bringing psychiatric attention to the potential for identifying persons at risk for genetic conditions such as Huntington disease, as well as confirming the genetic aspect of affective disorder, panic disorder, and others. And finally, the technology of the restriction fragment length polymorphism that identifies a marker for manic depressive disorder on chromosome 11 and on the X chromosome, thus documenting both the heterogeneity of inheritance in that condition and the potential for "reverse genetics" to find its pathologic characteristics. This last discovery, like many of the basic science observations in Osler's time, ends much of the argument about the cause of that condition.

In the midst of this list I do not want to miss the opportunity to emphasize how psychiatric clinicians put these new discoveries into place in a sophisticated manner. I could choose from many examples, but I would be less than human if I did not point out examples from my department of which I am quite proud and excited. My department has had a long interest in Huntington disease (McHugh & Folstein, 1975), and Dr. Susan Folstein has led an investigative team doing a survey of all people in Maryland with Huntington disease or at risk for it. The psychiatric issues of interest in that disease include the rather frequent appearance of manic-depressive disorder and an antisocial personality disorder in "at-risk" persons.

Most had assumed these psychiatric symptoms were psychological reactions to the at-risk plight. However, in a careful and clinically thoughtful epidemiologic study of these people that depended ultimately on her commitment to care for them in all their medical and psychological difficulties, Dr. Folstein showed that the manic-depressive disorder found in some families passed with the Huntington disease gene. Therefore, this psychiatric feature was an additional genetic burden linked to the etiologic agent. In practical terms, if an at-risk person displayed an intermittent depressive or manic disorder, it was almost certain that he or she would eventually show the deteriorating neurologic course.

In contrast, the appearance of antisocial personality in an at-risk person did not presage any greater likelihood of the neurologic disorder beyond the 50/50 chance that resided in the original at-risk status. The antisocial personality was not linked to the gene. Instead, Dr. Folstein identified it as a common outcome of a damaged family and disrupted childhood of these people, provoked by the destructive effect of Huntington disease on the capacities and conduct of their parents and the stability of their home.

Thus, from Huntington disease, Dr. Folstein has differentiated psychiatric syndromes distinct in their manifestations and quite distinct in their relationship to the disordered genome. One is directly linked to it; the other is an outcome indirectly tied to the gene through the sociocultural disorder it can produce in an instrument of personality formation—the family. I think it is obvious how all this information illuminates how we think not only about Huntington disease but about affective disorder and antisocial personality as well (Folstein et al., 1983).

Applications of This Pathway of Psychiatry

Why do I not simply point out events of modern psychiatry and avoid invidious comparisons across disciplines and departments? It is my point that these discoveries represent the products of a transition phase in psychiatry from a pre-Oslerian to a post-Oslerian discipline and, as most transition phases, they are, at the moment, awkward to fit into the traditional training and research programs of departments of psychiatry. When I speak of them to colleagues—both psychiatric and medical—I get similar and puzzled responses such as "Is that really psychiatric work," is it not "kind of neurological," or even once "you're a funny crowd there at Hopkins."

These attitudes are derived from a view of what a psychiatrist is—how he or she is identified as a psychiatrist—and regardless of the achievements and products of this new phase, this is a strictly pre-Oslerian issue. This attitude proposes that psychiatrists do psychotherapy and psychiatric patients have conditions susceptible to psychotherapy. It is this concept of a strict identification of psychiatrists with a particular treatment and restricted group of conditions which is the last hurdle to overcome in our passage through this transition phase into what I call post-Oslerian psychiatry.

Psychiatry is not synonymous with psychotherapy. Psychiatrists attend to and become expert in all disorders that manifest as changes in mental life regardless of the causes, mechanisms, or treatments. They thus share clinical and research interests with neurologists and internists on the one hand and with psychologists, sociologists, and other students of the human condition on the other, as well as have unique perspectives of their own. Clarity about this issue is crucial to our future. We must emphasize that a psychiatrist's domain of expertise embraces every disruption of mental life from mental retardation to dementia, from abnormal hungers to grief. Then we can show how information derived from knowledge of particular afflictions and from basic research can be programmatically deployed to teach medical students, residents, interested onlookers in other specialties, and, lest I forget, administrators, deans, and presidents of our university centers about the field. These people must be turned into active collaborators in the production of the emerging psychiatry; they will be enthusiastic for its new capacities if they can see where it is and the direction in which it is moving.

Let me specify the program of the future. It seems that an excessive emphasis on therapy and theories of therapy has hindered many educational programs in psychiatry, making too much of what is fundamentally too little. We must note the Oslerian directive and proceed in a fashion similar to the path medicine followed.

All psychiatrists must receive a solid education in the natural history of mental disorders. There must be emphasis, led by senior clinicians, on bedside and outpatient teaching where the basic features of each disorder can be exemplified, differentiating what is common to each condition from what is idiosyncratic to the patient at hand. This teaching should go on regularly in the form of rounds, clinical services, grand rounds, and journal club. Every psychiatrist should learn and relearn the particular signs and symptoms characteristic of every form of mental distress and disorder, separating one condition from another with as much confidence as possible at this time and with increasing reliability in the future. We must emphasize that progress depends on differentiation and that effective management and specific therapy emerges from differentiation and its comprehension.

At the same time, this education must teach the psychiatrist-in-training the relevant basic sciences and the related technology that illuminates aspects of these natural histories. For psychiatry, this basic knowledge must encompass not only physiology, pharmacology, epidemiology, and genetics but also psychology and sociology as they relate to abnormal human behavior. This can be achieved through seminars, lectures, minicourses, and supervised readings.

Psychiatrists must be versed and comfortable in discussing the more methodological aspects of the acquisition of knowledge about mental disorders. They do not have to become epistemologists, but they must be able to differentiate the empirical observations from meaningful interpretations in psychiatry, defining the appropriateness of both to advancing knowledge and appreciating the limits to an opinion restricted to either. This will discredit the overinflated generalizations of "pop psychology" that have mutilated our discourse. Observation, interpretation, practice, and research (essentially in that order) will progress together.

An education in science can be encouraged even more now because, like Osler, we psychiatrists are lucky in our time. The sciences that informed mental life in Osler's time were weak; now they have become powerful and illuminating. Their discoveries must become fundamental to all psychiatrists. Fortunately, the liveliness of those scientific disciplines is now expressed by many psychiatrists' interest, like many internists, in training themselves in both the clinical and the basic sciences. We also need texts like Osler's that emphasize the relationship of differentiated clinical conditions to scientific knowledge and do not exaggerate our contemporary treatment powers. At Hopkins, we have tried to write one (McHugh & Slavney, 1986).

What can we expect from this path? We can expect the results that Osler promised and delivered to medicine itself: an understanding of the differences among the patients we see and eventually an appreciation of the varieties of etiology and mechanism found in different psychiatric disorders. We can expect to realize preventive strategies and effective therapies based on this knowledge. But fundamentally, we can anticipate the emergence of a psychiatry identified by its subject matter, unified in its conceptual base, and no longer subdivided into camps with different "orientations."

Teaching and clinical work will go on in an atmosphere of research. This will lead to regular advances and more interprofessional collaboration. Psychiatry will bind itself more and more closely to medicine and will free itself from the politics of interpretative communities arguing with one another. It can bring to its students the excitement of progress and to its patients the best that devotion plus science can provide.

In this way, we will link up with the third of Osler's traditional heroes, Thomas Linacre, who instituted the Royal College of Physicians of London on letters patent from Henry VIII in 1518 in order to eliminate the indiscriminate practice of medicine in England, then being carried on by barbers, clergymen, and anyone else who felt inclined to take up the practice of medicine. (Do I need to note the similarity to the circus of psychotherapists today?) With the authority to examine and license physicians came the responsibility of placing medicine on an effective foundation and gradually freeing it from the idiosyncrasies that intermittently emerge in every human enterprise.

This time and this opportunity are now here for medicine's darling, psychiatry.

Annals of Internal Medicine, 1987

ACKNOWLEDGMENTS

The author thanks Gert H. Brieger and Marie Killilea for advice on earlier drafts of the paper and Susan Folstein for many discussions on Huntington disease.

Presented at the Annual Session of the American College of Physicians, 2 April 1987, New Orleans, on receipt of the William C. Menninger Memorial Award.

REFERENCES

Fleming, D. (1987). *William H. Welch and the rise of modern medicine.* Baltimore: Johns Hopkins University Press.

Folstein, S. E., M. L. Franz, B. Jensen, G. A. Chase, and M. F. Folstein. (1983). Conduct disorder and affective disorder among the offspring of patients with Huntington's disease. In *Childhood psychopathology and development,* ed. S. B. Guze, F. Earls, and J. E. Barrett, 231–245. New York: Raven Press.

Ludmerer, K. M. (1985). *Learning to heal: The development of American medical education.* New York: Basic Books.

McHugh, P. R., and M. F. Folstein. (1975). Psychiatric syndromes of Huntington's chorea: A clinical and phenomenological study: Seminars in psychiatry. In *Psychiatric aspects of neurologic disease,* ed. B. F. Benson and D. Blumer, 267–286. New York: Grune and Stratton.

McHugh, P. R., and P. R. Slavney. (1986). *The perspectives of psychiatry.* Baltimore: Johns Hopkins University Press.

Osler, W. (1895). Teaching and thinking: The two functions of a medical school. *Montreal Medical Journal* 23:561–572.

Psychiatry and Its Scientific Relatives

"A Little More Than Kin and Less Than Kind"

Psychiatry presents three special problems to all who wish to move the discipline forward as well as practice and teach it. The first is sectarianism, the almost cultic character of divisions within the discipline that proclaim one approach authentic and abuse others as "descriptive," "soft-nosed," or "moribund." The second problem is ambiguity over what distinguishes psychiatry from other specialties and secures its title to certain clinical conditions. If the specialty is to move forward, we had better know what it contains and why.

But the third and perhaps the most dismaying problem is the troubled discourse between psychiatry and the sciences that relate to it. In contrast to experimental medicine, in which the context of progress depends on a common vision of reality and an easy "two-way trade" of information between bedside and bench, behaviorists and neuroscientists are awkward allies of psychiatry despite their contributions. They hold with a philosophical tradition that poses ontological questions about mind, consciousness, and the self, proposing that these terms represent false beliefs and invalid "funny ways of talking." A scientific colleague who thinks that the conceptions that frame psychiatry's subject mattter are nonsensical, primitive, or incoherent can be a demoralizing companion but may be simply one who sees a different world and lives with a different set of problems than we do.

A sectarian field with an uncertain domain of responsibility flanked by sciences that occasionally deride its concepts is in deep trouble. The remedy for demoralization is always the same, however. Toughen up, clarify what *we* are and do, and discover how behaviorism and neuroscience can help us sometimes but can hinder us at others because of problems built into those views, some of which we are in a good position to identify but not all of which we have to accept.

Psychiatrists differ from other doctors by focusing attention on the domain of personal consciousness with its states, capacities, and behavioral potentials and its thoughts, moods, and perceptions. This "phenomenal world," to use the Gestaltist term, is acknowledged by all to be an awkward and ambiguous domain for study. It is fundamentally private, requiring a specialist's skill to approach and explore with confidence. But more crucial, its vivid personal qualities—percepts, beliefs, fears—seem untranslatable into the terms of brain and bodily structure on which they must depend. The mind/brain problem is critical to all who examine mental life because it presents a discontinuity within the hierarchical sequence of explanation (from mind down or brain up) that neither clinicians nor scientists have been able to eliminate.

The mind/brain problem provokes the concern of basic scientists with words such as consciousness and self. Their goal is the ultimate explanation of things. If such a word as *self* has qualities impossible to translate into physicochemical brain events, it may, like the terms tied to Ptolemaic astronomy or the flat-earth idea, become a distracting emphasis on "appearance" that obscures "realities" that are more fundamental.

Psychiatrists cannot wait for ultimate explanations. The mind/brain problem is a form of ignorance, but it is only one of several that burden them. Psychiatrists are doctors with a practical goal: apply to patients the *knowledge* that is available, in whatever terms it comes, and try to increase that knowledge by reflecting on that application. Founders of the discipline demonstrated how psychiatrists could scrutinize the mental state of patients and make discoveries that are helpful to science and practice, all without much concern over whether these were "appearances."

This pragmatic approach to the mind/brain problem that turns away from the conundrum to concentrate on the available knowledge about mental life does, however, impel other actions. It forces psychiatrists to describe how they organize their knowledge in ways that permit it to grow. It urges them to consider information from basic science for its help or hindrance to their efforts. With these actions, we psychiatrists become equal colleagues with basic scientists in the sense that we applaud their achievements, note their difficulties, and explain our own methods of reasoning and results.

Our methods have been described in a number of ways (dynamic, biological, systems theory, biopsychosocial, etc.). The approach that we (McHugh & Slavney, 1983) teach and find most compelling differentiates each method by its characteristic assumptions as a distinct "perspective" into the phenomenal world. Each perspective represents a generative viewpoint in the sense that it seizes upon certain observations and follows particular sequences of reasoning to produce an explanation of some aspect of mental life and its disorders. However, every perspective has "blind spots" to be revealed by other channels of knowledge (other perspectives) that emphasize other observations and follow different chains of logical assumptions to capture other aspects of the phenomenal world.

Behaviorists and neuroscientists provide information that can be used by psychiatrists. However, just how much help they provide varies from one perspective to another and from the very considerable to nil. I shall briefly describe the psychiatric perspectives, identify for each some of the contributions we get from the behavioral sciences and from the neurosciences, and finally approach open questions that still remain and should intrigue us all.

Psychiatrists use four distinct perspectives. The first is the *perspective of disease*, in which disorders in the phenomenal world, such as the collapse of cognitive capacities in dementia or the intrusion of abnormal experiences such as hallucinations, delusions, and fixed persisting mood states, are linked by the logic of correlation and categorical reasoning to abnormalities and distortions of brain structure or function. Discoveries in brain science from those accessible to the light microscope or the electroencephalogram to others resting upon new knowledge of receptor dynamics and neurochemical anatomy have gradually been correlated with psychological symptom clusters to validate the disease perspective as an illuminating approach to many psychiatric disorders. With, for example, the identification of a degeneration in the acetylcholine distribution system from the nucleus basalis in Alzheimer disease (Coyle, Price, & DeLong, 1983), the vista for new neuropathologies and their correlations with symptom groups seems almost unlimited. These achievements can be celebrated by psychiatrist and neuroscientist alike, as they collaborate in the disease perspective in ways identical to the collaboration of the other clinician-specialists with pathologists and basic scientists of all kinds.

The success of this collaboration and the fruitfulness of this perspective of disease for psychiatry prompt career development for individuals as both psychiatrists and neuroscientists. The disease perspective, however, although illuminating many disorders of the mind and applied whenever we speak of a dementia, delirium, manic-depressive disorder, and schizophrenia, does not explain all psychiatric problems or even all the symptoms of those with these diseases.

Some patients complain that they are distressed and overmastered by an intensity of feelings tied to motivated drives such as hunger, sexuality, or the cravings of addictions. It is not obvious that these patients have a unique qualitative alteration in mental state so much as that they are more powerfully driven by feelings common to all people. They sense problems in the excitation, inhibition, and regulation of these drives that may derive from many factors including past experience, present endogenous and exogenous stimuli, and efficiency of regulatory functions in the nervous system.

Psychiatrists approach these issues by a distinct perspective—the *perspective of behavior*—and describe the character of the cravings, their response to stimuli and inhibition, and the problematic outcomes that these disorders provoke. They entitle the disorders by the behavioral focus (e.g., alcoholism, pedophilia, bulimia, drug dependence). In understanding these conditions, psychiatrists seek help from neuroscientists and behaviorists. Thus, an appreciation of the links in brain and body to the motivations such as the regulatory function of sex hormones, the delineation of opiate receptor mechanisms, and the interaction of peripheral bodily states with central brain function in hunger has come to us from neuroscience. An appreciation of the reinforcements in the environment promoting addiction has come from behaviorism.

This again is an arena of achievement in the collaboration of neuroscience and behaviorism with psychiatry. It has promoted a major shift in psychiatric attention away from assuming that problems in motivated behaviors, such as those expressed in obesity and in distorted sexual cravings, have solely a symbolic meaning based on conflict. We now seek to identify brain-based mechanisms that generate behaviors and life experiences that shape them.

However, the science of motivation and drive is young. The neuroscience of motor sensory functions, for example, far outstrips it. Compare the sophisticated knowledge about the cellular organization of the cerebral cortex and the sequences of physiological events occurring within it to control arm movements (Evarts, 1981; Georgopoulis,

Schwartz, & Kettner, 1986) with our ignorance about the regulation of a particular behavior such as food intake, which might employ these very movements. We have scarcely a clue about what prompts a meal to start and precious little more about why it stops. Yet this would seem crucial behavioral and neuroscience-based information if we psychiatrists hope to derive a rational approach to bulimia, anorexia, or obesity, let alone to the large number of medical patients, such as those with cancer, whose loss of appetite exacerbates their illness.

We can say, "It is early times and help is on its way" (Goodwin, 1981). I certainly believe it—enough, after all, to attempt to hasten the day (McHugh & Moran, 1985); but I emphasize the dearth of information here not to be mean-spirited, pointing my finger at basic scientists, but to remind us all that the phenomenal world—the domain of psychiatric interest—is the domain where purpose reigns, and yet the brain mechanisms behind purpose are as unknown to neuroscience as to us.

Many patients seek psychiatric help not because they have abnormalities tied to disease, or because they are overmastered by the cravings of motivation, but because they find that they have difficulty meeting the demands of their life situations. They may be unable to comprehend what others can grasp easily. They are shy or uncertain in changing circumstances or too easily provoked by events into anxiety, hostility, depression, or risk taking.

Psychiatrists take a *dimensional perspective* here and propose that, just as people vary across the physical dimensions of height and weight, so they vary smoothly and quantitatively in dispositions, aptitudes, and inclinations. Individuals who deviate to an extreme along each dimension have difficulty in some circumstances—as the intellectually subnormal in school, the depressive introvert in planning the future, the "type A" personality in structuring social and leisure activities.

The recognition of these dimensions of variation, the reliability of their measurement, and their clinical utility has been a success story in psychiatry. Psychiatrists as venerable as Jung and Kretschmer have illuminated the role of dimensions in the appreciation of personality, and contemporary psychiatry has learned much from psychologists such as Eysenck, Costa, Meehl, and others about these issues.

There are problems in this perspective—mistakes and misuse of these ideas—just as each perspective needs refinement. Notice, however, that in contrast to the previous perspectives, neuroscience here has been essentially silent. I cannot point to a single neuroscience discovery that would explain the most obvious psychological differences among people. The brains of extroverts and those of introverts and even the brains of geniuses and those of the majority of persons with subnormal intelligence do not differ in any clear way. I know of no chemical, anatomical, or physiological function of the brain, inborn or developed, constitutional or environmentally provoked, that can be discerned to explain dimensional differences. The nervous systems seem remarkably uniform despite the most remarkable individual differences. The neuroscience explanations, as far as I know, remain submerged within the orders of magnitude that the billions of neurons and their connections permit.

But you might say, and I certainly would not disagree, "Give them a break." The neuron theory was only nailed down by Cajal some eighty years ago, distinctions in chemical anatomy discovered by Martha Vogt thirty-five years ago, and the columnar organization and the immensity of nerve numbers discovered by Mountcastle and Powell twenty years ago; work with receptor systems is so fresh that people are still arguing about credit! Explanations of dimensional characteristics will have to wait; but so far, nothing.

The final perspective psychiatrists use is the *perspective of the self and life story*. We choose this perspective for patients who come not because of disease, the intrusion of motivated drives, or deviation along some dimension of human variability but because they *intended* to do something—choose a job, sustain a marriage, succeed in college, relate to peers—and have suffered a number of unintended consequences: grief, isolation, demoralization, failure. They ask, "Where am I going and why can't I get there?" They are concerned with the results of their own actions. Here we confront the greatest challenge to the scientific foundations of our profession—selfness and intentionality.

People do not appear to be passive followers of their brain and body—and certainly no one thinks of him- or herself as such. Each self thinks that it is, to some extent, in charge of the body. "I" tell the brain what to focus on, not vice versa. The phenomenal world is a "willful" place: a place in which plans can be articulated, actions directed, and results appraised, criticized, or regretted. It is the domain of all the opposites, success and failure, virtue and vice, promises and betrayals. None of these can exist without selves, intentions, and life stories.

If it weren't such an everyday experience, it would be amazing. How does the material brain produce such a thing as the self and relate to it? How can we be true to mental life's material foundation without being false to the self's human capabilities and responsibilities?

When we psychiatrists look to basic scientists for help here, we get awkward, unsettling replies. It is not just that they cannot provide us with data-based answers; they seem to devalue the questions. The behaviorists promise blandly that knowledge yet to come of the reinforcements across a lifetime will explain all. Neuroscientists suggest indulgently that, because the characteristics of selfness identify a fundamental difficulty within the mind/brain problem, a preoccupation with the self is premature and may even be an expression of primitive thinking—a psychiatric romance, a dalliance with Descartes. These deferring responses are galling because they seem to scorn any serious attention to patent properties of mind and sources of mental disorder.

Some neuroscientists (Edelman and Mountcastle, 1978) do not deny the self and its prominent apparentness. They present information "from the bottom up" about the immensity of neuron numbers, the replication of identical multicellular modules in the cortex, and the numerous but selective interconnectivity among modules. They derive a concept of distributed systems with dynamic actions, accessible to both internally generated and externally induced neural activity. This is certainly a structural concept that approaches in complexity what would be needed for "selfness." Still, metaphors such as "image" and "readout" intrude in all this work and indicate that the leap from the brain up to the phenomenal world remains a leap across a gap unlike any other in the natural sciences. The phenomenal quality—the "I"-ness that is imaging and reading out—seems no closer even as the redundant mechanisms multiply and proliferate.

Equally, of course, "from the top down" it is difficult for the psychiatrist to see the link of the self, I-ness, to the brain. But that is an ancient problem. The bottom-up approach at least has the advantage of adding much information, even though we may not seem to be closer to the goal. In fact, as the remarkable anatomy and physiology of the brain emerge, the old chestnut for psychiatrists and psychologists is to wonder why, with natural selection, survival advantage might accrue to a system in which success or failure is illuminated by consciousness and felt by a self, rather than achieved automatically and unconsciously as by a programmatic functioning of the versatile and complicated machine neuroscience unveils. A mechanical way would certainly have saved much pain and suffering.

This is not simply a riddle for psychiatry. The neurophysiologist Charles Sherrington (1947) posed the same question and answered it by presuming that psychical elements must exert some influence on physical events, somehow enhancing the organism's power of disposing of its acts; but this is just another way of noting the apparent capacities of consciousness and the self, not explaining them, as he was quick to point out. Sherrington ended his introduction to his classic *The Integrative Action of the Nervous System* with the following statement: "That our being should consist of *two* fundamental elements offers I suppose no greater inherent improbability than that it should rest on one only" (1947, p. xx).

Few are prepared to make such a statement, and with perhaps the exceptions of John Eccles (1977) and Donald Griffin (1976), there may be no neuroscientist or behaviorist who is even thinking that way today. Yet I occasionally wonder what facts have been discerned since 1947 that would have made Sherrington change his mind if he had known them.

Many psychiatrists now think—and nothing as yet derived from behaviorism and neuroscience refutes the view—that there are open and free properties within human thought and self-generated, intentional behavior, properties that are not determined by external stimuli or internal physiological states. In this we are Cartesians, but unlike Descartes we cannot subscribe to an ultimate irreducibility of mind to brain. Most of us assume that science will eventually discover how the brain can deliver a directive self, intentionality, and the sense of vitality in the phenomenal world.

However, this discovery will not come about simply by a further accrual of the information we currently have but through a *revolution* in our understanding of properties that can spring into existence from neural systems and material. This revolution will bring an entirely new conception of the biological world and illuminate the place of freedom within it. The obliteration of the mind/brain gap demands something we do not imagine today, and if it occurs, none of us, neuroscientists, behaviorists, or psychiatrists (and citizens), will see the world as we do now.

But does how you think about the intractable mind/brain problem make any difference? I think it does. A sense that its solution will be revolutionary protects us from embracing the contemporary mechanistic determinism that would dim our view of that wonderful combination of freedom and constraint found in every healthy human being. Science may someday make this amalgam of brain and mind comprehensible. Surely such a revolution will amplify and dignify still further the work of psychiatry enhancing the freedom lost for people caught up in sickness and patienthood.

Journal of Nervous and Mental Disease, 1987

REFERENCES

Coyle, J. T., D. L. Price, and M. R. DeLong. (1983). Alzheimer's disease: A disorder of cortical cholinergic innervation. *Science* 219: 1184–1190.

Eccles, J. C. (1977). *The understanding of the brain.* New York: McGraw-Hill.

Edelman, G. M., and V. B. Mountcastle. (1978). *The mindful brain.* Cambridge, Mass.: MIT Press.

Evarts, E. V. (1981). Control of voluntary movement by the brain. In *Psychiatry and the biology of the human brain*, ed. S. Matthysse, 139–164. Amsterdam: Elsevier.

Georgopoulis, A., A. B. Schwartz, and R. E. Kettner. (1986). Neuronal population coding of movement direction. *Science* 233: 1416–1419.

Goodwin, D. W. (1981). Genetic component of alcoholism. *Annual Review of Medicine* 32:92–99.

Griffin, D. R. (1976). *The question of animal awareness.* New York: Rockefeller University Press.

McHugh, P. R., and T. H. Moran. (1985). The stomach: A conception of its dynamic role in satiety. *Progress in Psychobiological Psychology* 11:197–232.

McHugh, P. R., and P. R. Slavney. (1983). *The perspectives of psychiatry.* Baltimore: Johns Hopkins University Press.

Sherrington, C. (1947). *The integrative action of the nervous system.* New Haven, Conn.: Yale University Press.

A Structure for Psychiatry at the Century's Turn

The View from Johns Hopkins

I have three specific aims: first, to review some of the concepts supporting contemporary psychiatry in the United States; second, to explain the origins, strengths, and frailties of these particular foundations; and third, to provide examples of activity in the Department of Psychiatry at the Johns Hopkins School of Medicine that intends to both revise and restructure these foundations in ways that enhance teaching, practice, and research.

The Issues

Currently, much of American psychiatric practice rests upon undertakings launched in the late 1960s. The most celebrated achievement was the fashioning of a reliable approach to naming and classifying psychiatric disorders that culminated in the 1980 edition of the American Psychiatric Association's *Diagnostic and Statistical Manual of Mental Disorders* (DSM-III). This feat encouraged psychiatry programs to commit to research in a more collaborative and progressive spirit. As well, American psychiatrists seem to be abandoning allegiances to narrow explanatory theories about mental disorders. Many acknowledge a breadth of informative sources by enthusiastically supporting the encompassing "biopsychosocial" approach proposed by George Engel (1977, 1980).

DSM-III and the biopsychosocial concept settled some of the uneasiness in psychiatry provoked in the 1960s by growing appreciation of the unexpected and specific power of psychopharmacology, the awkward randomness in diagnostic practices, and the embarrassing "house divided" character of the discipline where "biologic" and "dynamic" factions contended. These new proposals had many features to recommend them. Each took a compromising stance toward contemporary practice and opinion. DSM-III admits to its canon any entity that can be "operationally" defined by its champions, and the biopsychosocial orientation seems ready to embrace any explanatory concept within its ample hierarchical arms.

The problems of these contemporary positions are not hard to find. In attempting to steer clear of the disputes that had riven psychiatry, the authors of DSM-III devised a classificatory system committed to empiricism. And empiricism for all its advantages at one stage in a discipline's growth is admittedly—and with DSM-III almost boastfully—a form of ignorance. By posing the existence of conditions DSM-III calls out for their validation and explanation. That call certainly encourages research, but DSM-III is a catalog, not a guide, and thus cannot recommend a path.

The biopsychosocial concept looks like the source of information to answer this call from DSM-III. The systems hierarchy (fig. 1) that Engel (1980) laid out reveals how restrictive any formulation of a clinical disorder would be if it were confined to matters *biologic, psychodynamic* or *social,* hence this term *biopsychosocial.* However, this approach is so broad in its scope and so nonspecific in its relation to any particular disorder that it can do no more than remind psychiatrists to be prepared to look at everything, and the interactions of everything, when seeking an explanation of any disorder. The biopsychosocial concept offers no rules, no directions, no logical pathways to explain the patient groupings in DSM-III. In this way, it is heuristically sterile. It provides ingredients but no recipes to specify the apt use of these ingredients in validating and explaining the categorically distinct disorders put forward in DSM-III.

In fact, the biopsychosocial idea is not new. It is quite simply Adolf Meyer's concept of psychobiology renamed and reanimated for the contemporary era. It retains all the strengths and limitations of that previous version. Meyer (1957) also embedded the person in a hierarchy of stratified systems ("interactive levels of integration" was his term) from the atom to the society (fig. 2). In proposing an explanation for any disorder, he encouraged a complete study of each patient's body, brain, and biography. Every mental disorder, he believed, stemmed from the responses of the person encountering the issues of a lifetime. He persuaded psychiatrists to seek within their "critical common sense," amply enhanced through this concept of integrative levels, the explanations and treatments of mental disorders.

Hierarchy of Natural Systems

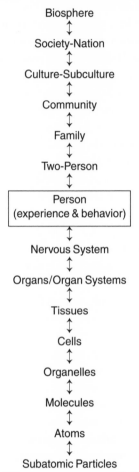

SYSTEMS HIERARCHY
(LEVELS OF ORGANIZATION)

Biosphere
⇅
Society-Nation
⇅
Culture-Subculture
⇅
Community
⇅
Family
⇅
Two-Person
⇅
Person
(experience & behavior)
⇅
Nervous System
⇅
Organs/Organ Systems
⇅
Tissues
⇅
Cells
⇅
Organelles
⇅
Molecules
⇅
Atoms
⇅
Subatomic Particles

Fig. 1. Engel's hierarchy. Reprinted from G. L. Engel (1980), with permission.

Meyer's energies derived from his opposition to simplicities and fatalistic implications that he discerned within the diagnostic and conceptual framework that came from Emil Kraepelin. He debunked the method of fixed-entity *diagnosis*, emphasizing instead individualized *formulations* for patients with mental illnesses.

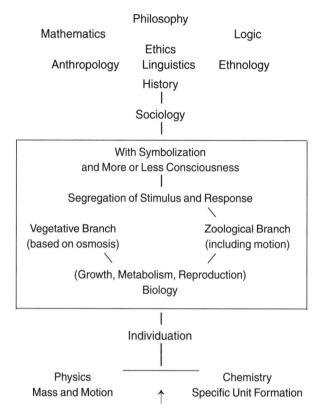

Fig. 2. Meyer's hierarchy. Reprinted from A. Meyer (1957), with permission.

It certainly was no coincidence that Engel's biopsychosocial concept, a restatement of Meyer's position, emerged into prominence in the same decade as DSM-III. It met and satisfied the same felt need as had its predecessor. Psychiatry in the United States is replaying a set of themes from earlier in this century. It is *both* neo-Kraepelinian and neo-Meyerian. But how these reappropriations of the past can steer our present activities into a more satisfactory future is not obvious.

A more thoroughgoing reappraisal of psychiatric explanations is required in the 1990s to answer the call from the neo-Kraepelinian DSM-III and yet sustain the ecumenical tenor of the neo-Meyerian biopsychosocial approach. Specifically we need a conceptual structure on which to rest an illuminating sequence of propositions about mental disorders and from which to derive a corresponding set of examples embodying and investigating these propositions.

A Structure for Explanations

We at Johns Hopkins hold that four standard methods for elucidating mental disorder are implicit (and should be made explicit) in contemporary psychiatric thought. We have called these methods four "perspectives" (McHugh & Slavney, 1983):

1. Disease perspective (the logic of categories)
2. Dimensional perspective (the logic of quantitation and individual variation)
3. Behavior perspective (the logic of teleology)
4. Life-story perspective (the logic of narrative)

We chose a visual metaphor because we wished to emphasize how each of these methods is a distinct viewpoint from which certain aspects of psychiatric disorders are clearly seen and others are obscured. In combination, they provide a basic structure for psychiatric explanations and illuminate what is pathologic in psychopathology.

Each perspective is rule-governed. Each is unique in its initiating premises, operational guidelines, logical sequences, and validating implications. Each, therefore, must be separately taught even though it may be employed with the others, in varying salience, in the elucidation of a particular clinical problem. Each perspective, because it reveals how we are thinking about certain disorders, enlarges what we know about all the patients in our care and enhances our grasp of what we are doing for them.

The *disease perspective* rests on a categorical logic. It attempts to cluster patients into separate groups, each group defined by the distinct features that are the defining characteristics of the disease. Embedded in the term *disease* is the implication that the ultimate and confirming characteristic endowing a patient with membership in a given category and distinguishing that patient from those in other categories will be an identifiable abnormality in structure or function of a bodily part.

The *dimensional perspective* applies the logic of quantitative gradation and individual variation to psychiatric disorder. It grapples with patients who cannot be placed in clear and distinct categories but can sometimes be comprehended in their vulnerability to mental distress from their individual position on psychological dimensions that are analogous to physical dimensions such as height or weight.

The *behavior perspective* emphasizes the goal-directed, often goal-driven, teleologic aspect of human activities. It notes that disorders can emerge either because of the abnormal goals some people can come to crave (as in drug addiction) or because of an excess in their attempts to satisfy drives common to all (as in eating to obesity).

Finally, the *life-story perspective* rests on the logic of narrative. It draws on the occurrence of events in the patient's past to understand his or her current distress, and more specifically, it posits the existence of a piloting self whose choices somehow bring about unintended consequences, all illuminated by the persuasive power of narrative.

Notice that we do not describe a "biologic" or a "dynamic" perspective. Biologic and dynamic issues figure in each of our perspectives but vary in salience from the disease to the life-story perspective in an almost reciprocal fashion. Also, just as we do not find it helpful in teaching this structure for psychiatric explanations to specify a separate neurophysiologic perspective, or a sociologic perspective, or a psychopharmacologic perspective, so we do not put forward a separate developmental perspective. Development, like physiology and like culture, is everywhere. Thus in our proposal it forms an ingredient (an important ingredient, admittedly) for each of these perspectives rather than a perspective itself.

Disease Perspective

The logic of this perspective is a categorical one. It rests upon the fact that signs and symptoms of some disorders tend to cohere in recognizable clusters or syndromes that progress in characteristic ways. The elucidating chore is driven by the need to explain this cohesion. Once physicians recognize a group of patients with a distinctive cluster of symptoms, they begin to wonder whether a bodily pathology (either in structure or function) and a biologic etiology might be provoking the condition. Successful discoveries of these latter elements confirm both the opinion that the clinical category is appropri-

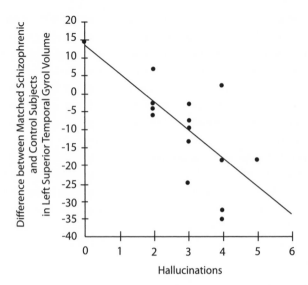

Fig. 3. Increasing auditory hallucinations as left superior temporal gyrus shrinks in schizophrenic subjects with respect to matched controls. Reprinted from P. E. Barta et al. (1990), with permission.

ately considered a disease and the embedded implication that its nature rests on a disruption of bodily mechanisms. Psychiatrists treat many confirmed diseases (dementia, delirium etc.) without quarreling about whether the concept is appropriately applied to them.

Both computerized axial tomography (CAT) and magnetic resonance imaging (MRI) have shown that brains of schizophrenic patients often have atrophy implying damage. Among the best examples of such work are the studies of identical twins discordant for schizophrenia of Suddath et al. (1990), where these clear distinctions between the normal and the abnormal subjects are evident in their brain images.

At Johns Hopkins, Barta et al. (1990) demonstrated not only evidence of atrophy in the left superior temporal gyrus but also a clear correlation of this atrophy with the severity of the hallucinatory experiences in their patients with schizophrenia (fig. 3). This is some evidence confirming that schizophrenia will, like epilepsy, emerge as a product of brain pathology and that its particular symptoms, of which hallucinatory experiences are but one, may be linked to distinct sites of damage in the brain.

This work is but beginning. I admire it because it neatly exemplifies what is expected when employing the disease perspective to elucidate a mental disorder. Symptoms are linked to pathology and a search for etiologies—which, for schizophrenia, may be of several kinds (birth injury, anoxia, genetic vulnerability, etc.)—can be launched. If this research program is successful in its search for causes, then rational treatment and prevention become possible.

Yet everyone knows that *disease* is not an appropriate term for all distress or difficulty. To teach that all disorders are kinds of disease will misconstrue matters of importance in practice and research, implying as it does that neuroscience will provide an anomalous neuron for every anomalous thought.

Dimensional Perspective

Psychological dimensions with their logic of gradation and quantitation provide a contrast to disease. There are several psychological features across which humans vary in a graded fashion much as they vary in such physical characteristics as height and weight. An individual who deviates to an extreme along such a dimension can, under certain circumstances, suffer because of it.

Individual variation is as apparent in affective characteristics as it is in cognitive characteristics such as intelligence. Axis II of DSM-III attempts to capture this variation within categories or typologies (histrionic, narcissistic, compulsive, etc.) and thus follows a pattern of reasoning similar to that used with disease. At Johns Hopkins, we agreed that the features defining these types in DSM-III are unlike the symptoms of disease in their all being graded phenomena. We proposed an approach that assessed such features in a dimensional fashion as with intelligence assessment. We believed that the results would display the nature of certain clinical conditions more clearly than does the categorical approach.

If, as with intelligence, the distressed individuals seen as patients in hospitals and clinics represent those people toward one extreme on a dimension of variation, then a population-based survey would be needed as the source of basic data for dimensional reasoning. We tackled this task in the local Baltimore population, among our contributions to the National Epidemiologic Catchment Area (ECA) study.

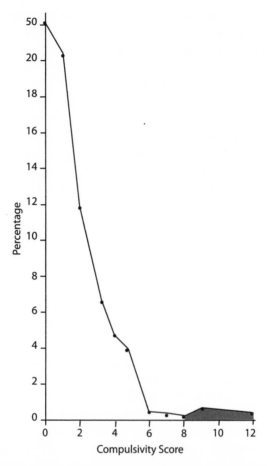

Fig. 4. Prevalence (%) of compulsive features in the Baltimore population and (shaded) the prevalence and position on this compulsivity scale of subjects who satisfied DSM-III criteria for compulsive personality disorder. Reprinted from G. Nestadt et al. (1991), with permission.

Here I shall discuss the findings for the compulsive personality disorder (Nestadt et al., 1991). Five features, says DSM-III, constitute the characteristics of that disorder: indecision, stubbornness, work devotion, perfectionism, and emotional constriction. The striking aspect of the results of this research is how many people in Baltimore have some compulsive features and how the individuals who satisfy the DSM-III criteria for the compulsive personality disorder are the minority at the extreme on the dimension (fig. 4).

This observation could be an outcome of the methods employed in the study, but a validating set of assessments were available to test whether the actual score on this scale of compulsivity could identify either a risk for certain conditions or a protection from others. This is exactly what emerged when the DSM-III conditions, generalized anxiety disorder (GAD), and alcohol disorders, were correlated with the compulsivity score. There was a clear enhancement of risk for GAD as the score increased and a clear protection against alcoholism in an almost "dose-response" fashion.

My major point here is simple. A dimensional perspective illuminates some psychiatric disorders better than does the more strictly categorical logic tied to disease reasoning. It is compatible with the sense of individual variation in disposition that is familiar to every psychiatrist making a personality diagnosis. Finally, it brings into focus a substrate of risk and protection that is comprehensible for elucidating other psychiatric disorders.

Behavior Perspective

The idea I wish to communicate with the term *behavior* is the significance of the goal-directed aspect of many human actions. Disorders of human behavior may rest either on disrupted bodily mechanisms—as in hypothalamic obesity—or on culturally induced goals such as the "sick" role sought in hysteria. Many clinically significant behaviors probably derive from both life experience and embodied mechanisms. Drug addictions or various sexual abnormalities are examples in which both the inducements and enticements of a persuasive public may provoke the first act of what then becomes a behavioral pattern self-sustained by a craving derived from both pharmacophysiology and conditioning. Once the concept of the behavior perspective is appreciated, an approach radically different from the disease perspective recommends itself for the treatment of these disorders. The initial focus of treatment is to use every measure to *stop* the behavior—a kind of "symptomatic" approach that would be scorned as superficial in the management of disease.

Behaviors tend to be self-sustaining for many reasons: the bodily toxicities associated with drug abuse prompt repetition of drug-taking behavior; changes in the social network provoked by illness-imitating hysterical behavior may encourage it; starvation's disruption to bodily and psychological integrity in anorexia nervosa renders the patient inaccessible to counsel. These issues are magnified by the habit aspect that derives from simple recurrence of behavior and encourages it.

All the programs for behavior disorders (anorexia nervosa, alcoholism, sexual disorder) at Johns Hopkins share the opinion derived from this perspective that treatments for such conditions must be staged. The starting point is always a major effort to stop the behavior, and if pharmacologic measures can help, they are employed. Throughout the course of treatment efforts are made to ensure that the behavior does not recur. Only once the behavior is stopped can therapy successfully move on to the later steps such as treating comorbid disorders (depression, anxiety, etc.), elucidating vulnerabilities of temperament, deconditioning, and addressing habit-sustaining social attitudes.

Finally, it is as behaviors that linkages to basic science will emerge for these conditions. For example, at Johns Hopkins we have been active in attempting to curtail the craving for drugs that sustains the behavior of addiction. The investigators in our Behavioral Pharmacology Research Unit (BPRU) have combined approaches that attempt to combat the operant conditioning features sustaining drug abuse (Stitzer, Bigelow, & Gross, 1989) with research on the clinical application of new medications to suppress the rewards of drug-seeking and drug-taking activities. Recent work at the BPRU has focused on buprenorphine (Bickel et al., 1988a, b), a compound with both opiate agonist and antagonist features, thus combining aspects found in methadone and naloxone. It may prove to be an ideal compound to help patients stop opiate abuse, particularly if it is integrated into a program of behavioral management as advocated by the BPRU (Stitzer, Bigelow, & Gross, 1989).

Life-Story Perspective

The final perspective—and for some the one most identified with psychiatrists—is that of the life story. It presumes that distressing mental states can be the outcome of a series of self-involved life events and these events are best depicted when presented in a narrative form. The fundamental component of the clinical story, like any personal narrative depicting a result, is how setting, sequence, and a self's intentional interactions can make a seemingly chaotic mental state the understandable outcome of the wishes and wants of the individual.

The life-story perspective can be a part of any formulation including those formulations that rest on the disease, dimensional, or behavioral perspectives. In fact, it could be said that in all distress or disorder, some aspect of the individual's life story provides understanding to elements of the clinical presentation. But a story can be the primary way of comprehending a state of distress.

This method of elucidating a mental disorder by describing a coherent role for the patient in its generation (adding ingredients from the dynamic unconscious if needed) can promote therapeutic optimism and confidence in both the patient and the psychiatrist. If the condition is in part derived from the self's intentions and motives—especially ones that need unearthing—then reconstructed, conscious intentions can set in motion new life plans, sequences, and more satisfactory outcomes. The story is the major basis of psychotherapy and transmits an excitement encouraging patient care.

A missionary fervor, however, may develop around the story method and is often at the heart of the conflict between various schools of dynamic psychiatry. Thus Freudians propose that hidden libidinal conflicts should be sought to illuminate manifest disorder, while Adlerians claim that power drives are at the root of things and need to be brought to light and rescripted. Each school of psychotherapy tends to produce version after version of the same story despite the different ingredients of person, place, and time in their patients.

The insistence upon retelling the same story suggests a dogmatic commitment or gnostic zeal ("we know the secret") that transforms teaching into initiation. A subliminal awareness of this feature is an issue for most young psychiatrists. It repels some and draws others into segregated training institutes. In all, it produces an uneasiness over their educational pathway that can be dispelled only by recognizing its source within the life-story perspective.

At Johns Hopkins, the research of Jerome Frank has done much to relieve this problem by turning the customary therapeutic and elucidatory aspects of the life-story perspective around. He demonstrated, from looking at the patients treated by psychotherapists, that what they share is not their stories but their states. This state he described well as "demoralization." It can derive from many different circumstances and life sequences.

This view of Frank's directed his research into the commonalities of psychotherapies rather than their differences. In the most recent edition of his impressive book *Persuasion and Healing* (Frank & Frank, 1991), he and his coauthor, Julia Frank, repeatedly display how the illumination from quite distinct "story lines" can bring recovery to demoralized individuals. The key to psychotherapy is not the elucidation of the "correct" story. Help emerges from the patient's sense that he or she is understood by some authority who is prepared to provide assistance in restructuring his or her thoughts and intentions into a story with more promising meanings. This can restore a sense of mastery of life critically absent from the initial demoralized state.

Thus, the life stories, which have been so illuminating and yet so divisive in psychiatry, have been reemphasized in a radically different way. We see commonalities in outcome more than commonalities to the story lines. We appreciate that the great theorists have provided a collection of themes for our consideration. We can select the most appropriate themes for the narrations we draw with our patients, ones that fit the particular situation and do not depend upon some esoteric, sectarian knowledge of something hidden in human nature.

Resolution

I have attempted three things. First, I discussed some contemporary foundations of psychiatry in the United States to show their merits but also how they are recurrent notions that now, as in their previous appearances, leave much unresolved. Second, I wished to propose a set of elucidating and encompassing perspectives that can, when made explicit, restructure our thought. Each perspective has its own logic, grapples with certain psychiatric issues most naturally, and yet can be coordinated with the other perspectives in practice. Finally, I tried to review briefly a current application of each perspective at Johns Hopkins so as to show how every one of them can be embodied in teaching, practice, or research.

We are all challenged to find ways to assimilate the amorphous body of psychiatric fact and opinion. This is the response from Hopkins. The effort is to entrench our professional claims and competences on what we know and how we know it, dispelling both the caprice that emboldens pop psychology and the mystery that kindles faction. We should demonstrate not only that we are a part of medicine but also how we are a vital and distinctive part with a *structured* body of knowledge unique to us as specialists.

Journal of the Royal Society of Medicine, 1992

ACKNOWLEDGMENTS

The lecture was dedicated to Sir Aubrey Lewis, in the happy memory of my days as a Research Fellow at the Institute of Psychiatry under his supervision in 1960/61. I thank Patrick Barta, George Bigelow, Jerome Frank, Gerald Nestadt, Godfrey Pearlson, Alan Romanoski, and Maxine Stitzer for helping me see more deeply into their work. I thank Marie Killilea, Timothy Moran, and Phillip Slavney for their helpful suggestions on the manuscript. This work was supported by the Lorraine and Leonard Levin Research Fund and grants # DK 19302 and # MH 15330 from NIH. None of it would even have been thought but for conversations held on Ward Seven with James Gibbons, Gerald Russell, and Ted Smith all those years ago.

REFERENCES

Barta, P. E., G. D. Pearlson, R. E. Powers, S. S. Richards, and L. E. Tune. (1990). Auditory hallucinations and smaller superior temporal gyral volume in schizophrenia. *American Journal of Psychiatry* 147:1457–1462.

Bickel, W. K., M. L. Stitzer, G. E. Bigelow, I. A. Liebson, D. R. Jasinski, and R. E. Johnson. (1988a). A clinical trial of buprenorphine: Comparison with methadone in the detoxification of heroin addicts. *Clinical Pharmacology and Therapeutics* 43:72–78.

——. (1988b). Buprenorphine: Dose-related blockade of opioid challenges effects in opioid dependent humans. *Journal of Pharmacology and Experimental Therapeutics* 247:46–53.

Engel, G. L. (1977). The need for a new medical model: A challenge for biomedicine. *Science* 196:129–136.

——. (1980). The clinical application of the biopsychosocial model. *American Journal of Psychiatry* 137:535–544.

Frank, D. D., and J. D. Frank. (1991). *Persuasion and healing: A comparative study of psychotherapy*. 3rd ed. Baltimore: Johns Hopkins University Press.

McHugh, P. R., and P. R. Slavney. (1983). *The perspectives of psychiatry*. Baltimore: Johns Hopkins University Press.

Meyer, A. (1957). *Psychobiology*. Ed. E. E. Winters and A. M. Bowers. Springfield, Ill.: Charles C Thomas.

Nestadt, G., et al. (1991). DSM-III compulsive personality disorder: An epidemiological survey. *Psychological Medicine* 21:461–471.

Stitzer, M. L., G. E. Bigelow, and J. Gross. (1989). Behavioral treatment of drug abuse. In *Treatments of psychiatric disorders*, vol. 2. Washington, D.C.: American Psychiatric Association.

Suddath, R. L., G. W. Christison, E. F. Torrey, M. F. Casanova, and D. R. Weinberger. (1990). Anatomical abnormalities in the brains of monozygotic twins discordant for schizophrenia. *New England Journal of Medicine* 322:789–794.

Treating the Mind as Well as the Brain

A mini-rebellion broke out last summer in psychiatry, perhaps the most disputatious of all medical disciplines. The current rebels are demanding changes in the official handbook—the fourth edition of the American Psychiatric Association's *Diagnostic and Statistical Manual of Mental Disorders* (1994), known as DSM-IV, which lists the conditions that the association designates as disorders (and that health insurance companies will pay psychiatrists for treating). The rebels want to add to that list a category called relational disorders, which would encompass the emotional and behavioral distress that can emerge through misunderstanding between such partners as husband and wife, or parent and child.

The psychiatric association rejects the rebels' proposal, arguing that contemporary psychiatry views mental illnesses as linked to brain disorders in the same way that other medical specialties, like cardiology, link the conditions they study to disorders in bodily organs. Relational disorders defy that medical model because only an individual, not a relationship, can have a sick brain.

But the idea that the only real psychiatric disorders are those tied to brain defects—an idea sometimes expressed by the slogan "for every twisted thought, its twisted neuron"—is incoherent in both philosophy and application.

First, the philosophy: of course, nothing happens in mental life without brains. The brain is the source of our thinking, including our hopes, our fears, our ups, our downs. Everything that could be considered psychological—both normal and abnormal—is produced by the neurobiological capacities of the brain. But the conclusion that every mental disorder derives from brain disorder oversimplifies a profound matter.

All consciousness comes from the brain, but consciousness interacts with the brain that generates it in a special, as yet inexplicable, way. The conscious mind gives a personal, privately sensed direction to the brain's activity. Although how subjective thought can direct the objective activity of the brain puzzles scientists, the implication is that some mental disorders derive from brain deficits and others from personal thoughts and decisions.

Specifically, the conscious mind is not a product of the brain in the same way that urine is a product of the kidney, or bile a product of the liver. Those bodily products offer no mysteries to science today. Their sources are clear and their utility obvious. But the conscious mind, although just as surely a biological product, causes subsequent activity in the bodily organ—the brain—from which it emerges.

A mindless world would work automatically. The mind-full world, as we know from direct experience, works with choices, reasons, plans, hopes—all perceived as "mine." With the freedom produced by consciousness, we have the makings of happiness and sadness—and, of course, of good and ill.

Consciousness is an interactive property of brain life, with both bottom-up and top-down aspects. Brains bring about consciousness (bottom up), but consciousness leads brain activity to follow its designs (top down).

We know that interaction as plainly as we know ourselves. But neuroscientists have no conception of how the brain operates to produce or relate to consciousness as we experience it. The mind/brain problem remains a fundamental enigma to science.

Psychiatrists cannot and should not wait for the solution to that problem—nor should they prejudge its character, as the medical model of psychiatry does. They must identify and treat mental problems that come from the bottom up, the top down, or both together. One group is no more real than another.

Bottom-up problems are easier to understand because they derive from physical ailments like infectious diseases or vascular strokes, which break down the brain just as similar afflictions damage or destroy other organs. The indication in consciousness of a disruption of the underlying brain will be the appearance of symptoms like dementia or hallucinations. Broken brain parts bring about broken mental faculties. Psychiatrists, along with neurologists and other brain scientists, can link the brain damage to the character and extent of those deformations of mind—from the bottom up—and then work to cure them.

Top-down mental disorders do not emerge as deformations of mental faculties but as emotional and behavioral responses—quite normal in their character but causing distress in their quality and degree—to unexpected or unwelcome results of the conscious mind's assumptions, plans, and choices. With our freedom to choose, we can get into serious trouble even when our brain machinery works properly. Our conscious mind determines whether we behave in a way that disappoints our friends and leads to painful feelings of embarrassment and shame, or behave in a way that makes others admire us.

Top-down disorders are dysfunctional rather than deformational. They bring demoralization, anger, and resentment from frustrated intentions and desires. The brain supports the intentions and registers the distress, but conscious thought is responsible for choosing the intentions. Only better thought and planning will lead to recovery.

With top-down disorders, psychiatrists work as teachers or coaches to conscious agents, not as apothecaries or nerve mechanics. The object of that psychiatric effort is to illuminate a patient's situation, mature or enrich his or her goals in life, and help him or her see how to achieve them.

Bottom-up and top-down aspects of consciousness can interact in some clinical situations. Specifically, a bottom-up affliction like Alzheimer disease or bipolar disorder will also—by its consciously appreciated implications for the future—provoke top-down fears, worries, and concerns. That explains why such conditions call for both medications and psychotherapy: medications for the bottom-up symptoms, and therapy for top-down anxieties.

So much for the philosophy behind psychiatry's medical model; how about its application? Patients with either deformational (bottom-up) or dysfunctional (top-down) disorders go to a psychiatrist because they want an expert to identify their trouble and prescribe a treatment. To say that only the deformational disorders are really psychiatric—and thus to presume that the dysfunctional disorders either are not disorders at all or are deformational disorders in disguise—is folly. Any distressing mental state or behavior that causes a patient to seek help from a psychiatrist is a real disorder.

Relational disorders are real in just that sense, and a manual of psychiatric diagnoses should include them. They are common complaints of people who come to psychiatrists for treatment. They rest on misapprehensions and misunderstandings between partners in a relationship and generate much mental distress. But they respond well to treatment when a therapist guides both parties to reframe their habits and adapt more accommodating demeanors. With such top-down treatment, the brains of both individuals distressed by the relational problem will change—but through conscious reflection and redirection, not through manipulations of brain tissue. Contemporary claims that psychotherapy works directly on the brain ignore the intervening role of consciousness and its top-down power.

The mini-rebellion of the summer of 2002 may encourage the American Psychiatric Association to abandon its stubborn commitment to an untenably rigid medical model. That welcome change would underline what psychiatrists agree about: the mind is a phenomenon of life, actively involved in health and affliction, derived from and yet guiding neurobiological activity. It would also help bring about a classification of psychiatric disorders that reflects the clinical implications of the interaction between the mind and the brain.

The Chronicle of Higher Education, 2002

Part V

VISTAS AND VIEWS

Finally, what can psychiatrists say that might bring insight into issues outside the clinic? Does their expertise extend beyond patient services or not? I, like many of my brethren, am prone to claim some powers but warn that perhaps what we know and how we know it permit us to offer here only guiding suggestions, not directives or prescriptions.

Even with such qualifying remarks, though, we may provide some insights to others. After all, Freud was as sought after as Einstein for his opinions on Western culture and took that as encouragement to comment extensively about everything from artists such as Leonardo to religious leaders such as Moses himself. All of civilization seemed to him at least within his conceptual grasp.

I lack the confidence of the lofty Freud but have occasionally given way to the impulse of describing what a psychiatrist notices in matters of interest to the public. This part of the book contains several essays and lectures prompted either by questions asked of me or by the spontaneous energy of an impulse. I think for the most part I'm trying to transmit some knowledge and encourage prudence in its application given the "mountains" of doubt remaining for students of the mind.

I'm averse to offering "keys" to the "deep" forces behind our lives and tend to a realist's view that asks "What can be seen, what can be sensed, and what can be done on the basis of public information?" This theme if faithfully employed does bring about some enthusiasm for study and discussion of the place of psychiatry outside the clinic.

Two Perspectives on Consciousness

I want to thank the Loyola chapter of Phi Beta Kappa for inviting me to address its new members and the university community. The honor is redoubled by the recollection of my own induction day at another college when my dear father accompanied me during the ceremonies. His witness to such a tangible event as my election to this honorable fraternity confirmed for him that I had not wasted the many efforts he had devoted to my benefit and gave us both deep satisfaction. I think of that day as one of the times—far fewer than they should have been—when I thanked him in a most direct fashion. Thus, this day is both an honor and a recapture of one of my most heartfelt experiences.

But I was not invited to reminisce about my youth, happy though it was. I was invited to talk to you—briefly I was instructed—about what I have grasped in my maturity that might be of interest on an occasion when your demonstrated capacities to learn are celebrated and when your future is being contemplated.

I presume I was invited because I am a psychiatrist who studies severe mental illnesses. Thus, before I start on my main theme, let me disabuse any of you who think that as a psychiatrist I know the secrets of life and have brought them with me to Loyola today. Psychiatrists work with mental disorder, and as a result we know a lot about what gets people down but little or nothing about what makes people great. We, like everyone else, are struck dumb with admiration by heroes and heroines, big and small, noted and unnoted, living and dead. And we have little or no idea what made them what they are beyond the kinds of devotion you have shown in your own efforts here at Loyola over the past several years.

Psychiatrists are physicians. We work in clinics with the handicapped. We do good work and help many people to recover. But we don't explain courage, endurance, commitment, creativity, or any of the other vigorous virtues exemplified among your group of scholars. One should no more expect a psychiatrist working in a clinic to explain, say, the remarkable achievements of Ignatius Loyola than expect an orthopedist who works on broken joints and bones to explain the grace, fortitude, and athleticism of Cal Ripken or Kristi Yamaguchi. We fix them when they're hurt but they do their thing on their own.

If I can't give you the secrets of life because I do not know them, what can I do? And it was that question that prompted my title—"Two Perspectives on Consciousness." Because if there is one thing I do know something about, it's human consciousness. It is within consciousness that psychiatrists seek manifestations of disorder, just as dermatologists seek disorders in the skin and cardiologists seek disorders in the heart. I hope to explain to you just what I mean by consciousness, why it is an intriguing domain of life, all primarily to describe how in my experience there emerged, within communities where I do most of my work, an intriguing but dislocated set of attitudes—now resolving—about the nature and purpose of the conscious experience, attitudes that tend to downplay its contingency and its freedom.

By consciousness I mean subjective experience, the experience of our own thoughts, perceptions, and feelings as those features belong to our inner selves—the painfulness of pain, the redness of red, the delightfulness of love, the reflectiveness and successions of thought, the discomfiture and drive of hunger, and ultimately the me-ness of me in action. In this sense consciousness is the most immediate of our experiences—that of which we are most certain. Consciousness impresses itself upon us at every waking moment and intermittently in dreams during sleep. In fact, there is nothing I am more sure of than my consciousness—much more sure of it than that any of you here are conscious of me.

And yet if there is a bigger mystery in the natural sciences than consciousness, I don't know it. This essential aspect of our life eludes explanation. We know consciousness is the product of our brain because various kinds of treatments that alter the brain can either alter consciousness, as in intoxications, or occlude it altogether, as in general anesthesia. However, we do not know how the brain produces these special experiences of subjective awareness. This issue is referred to as the mind-brain problem.

You can read many books and treatises on this subject—many I've found of considerable interest—but let me spare you some effort right now by saying that after you read these books, fascinating as they are, you will know one simple fact: we do not have a clue how a material object—even one as complicated as our brain—can produce the light of consciousness in which we experience our thoughts, carry out our enterprises, and in so many different ways conduct our lives. Everyone agrees that the brain is necessary for consciousness, but, in the end, no one can explain how it is sufficient given what we know about our mental powers.

This unresolved problem lies at the heart of how issues of consciousness separate the opinions of two groups with whom I've worked during my career—two related but essentially distinct groups of colleagues.

Half of the time, I work in laboratories with physiologists and neuroscientists attempting to understand the brain and body mechanisms tied to behavior. The other half I work in clinics with a variety of therapists of human mental and behavioral disorders. Both groups, neuroscientists and therapists, understand the mind/brain problem but—most intriguingly—differ sharply on its implications.

In describing their differences one tends to stumble toward the cliché of "two cultures," but that would be quite wrong. These two groups belong to the same culture—the contemporary university in a liberal, pluralistic society. However, they differ seriously over consciousness and what to make of it.

The neuroscientists, because of their interest in reducing mind to brain, are suspicious—sometimes to the point of contempt—of much "mind" talk, suspecting that behind such talk is an effort to introduce ghosts into the machinery of the nervous system. And yet these very scientists believe that through the contents of their consciousness— their thoughts, perceptions, and insights—they can move toward truth and an accurate impression of reality. All therapists unapologetically discuss mind and matters conscious. However, many of them insist that consciousness is untrustworthy because its contents —the same thoughts, perceptions, and insights on which scientists depend—are actually distortions and illusions rather than reflections of reality. These attitudes, both those of suspicion and those of allegiance, differentiate these two groups tied to psychiatry.

Let me develop these distinctions and explain what I have come to make of them. When you speak to many neuroscientists—not all, to be sure, but many—you discover that they can become witheringly scornful during almost any discussion of some commanding role for consciousness in nature and over the brain. They intend to replace what they view as speculations about consciousness and its authority with observations on brain states—bottom up rather than top down, as they might express it. They believe that a preoccupation with consciousness, for itself, can be "soft" science, if science at all. They will grumble about "folk psychology" if you mention the self or the subjective world of consciousness. The toughest among them may say such things as "science shows there is no soul" and then classify your views about these matters with the cosmological beliefs of primitive tribes and nomads who populated the heavens with spirits and presumed a geocentric rather than a heliocentric planetary system. You may be considered one small step from the "flat-earth" crowd.

On the other hand, for themselves, neuroscientists hold that consciousness—consisting, as I said, of subjective appreciation of the working thoughts and perceptions—is their source of intelligibility, for making sense of the world that exists outside consciousness. Through thinking and observing they have come to believe that the universe is one of order and that, by thinking hard about it, they can discern that order—and discover its fundamental features. They believe that by working over their thoughts they will identify more powerful, more predictive, more control-enhancing, and indeed more truthful ways of viewing nature. By the conscious activity of thinking, they progress.

Indeed, most scientists endow thinking about a problem (a subjective, private feature of consciousness) with more respect than they endow technical skill applied to a problem (an objective, observable activity). Thus they know that technical skill may be necessary to work out the mechanics of flight or the cure for a disease but such skill cannot replace mental ingenuity—mind work—which directs these skills.

A neat example of my point is an admiring, almost envious, description of James Watson, the discoverer of the structure of DNA, by another Nobel laureate, Max Perutz, quoted by Horace Judson in his magisterial book *The Eighth Day of Creation* (1979). Perutz said, "[F]or Jim's [scientific problem] there was an elegant solution. . . . He found it partly because he never made the mistake of confusing hard work with hard thinking; he always refused to substitute the one for the other. Of course, [that gave him] time for tennis and girls."

How different this homage to thought from the doubting neuroscientists is from many therapists' attitudes about consciousness. In contrast to neuroscientists, therapists do not dismiss consciousness. They never speak of "folk psychology" or disparage reflections on inner life. They know that consciousness is real and—up to a point—they are prepared to give credence to the power of subjective thoughts, feelings, and attitudes.

What therapists doubt, often with mocking skeptical disdain, is that consciousness is trustworthy. They hold that most people's ideas are manifest distortions of reality, illusions produced by unacknowledged, self-serving wishes and impulses. Many therapists, perhaps overly influenced by their experiences in clinics, will say that most people's "points of view"—the voiced expressions of consciousness— are neurotic rationalizations, political defenses of vested interests, or some other self-justifying, socially generated compulsion to misrepresent the truth to themselves.

Although I, as a therapist, agree that the thoughts and attitudes of patients need correction, what I wish to deny is that consciousness is naturally misdirected, a mask for defensive selfishness, or a distorting mirror on the truth for us all. In fact, consciousness often provides an experience so insistent, so telling, and so truthful that its message about reality is as emphatic as a punch in the nose.

A woman once came to see me because, as she said, she was miserable and wondered if I could help her with some medications. She then told me that her husband had been killed in an auto accident three months before. When I, rather promptly, tied this event to her misery, she explained that her friends and a therapist had told her that she "should be over it" because three months of grief was morbid and perhaps self-serving.

My response was to say that she had silly friends and that there was nothing morbid in the duration of her sadness but that it honored, instinctively, the reality of her affection and her loss. I would not give her medication but would help her see that she had been "mugged by consciousness," hit by what counts in life, and so learned of the powers to truth embedded in our natures.

To summarize, many neuroscientists, for all that they appreciate their own consciousness, when queried about its nature, reject the concept of conscious control of their brains with which they function. Many therapists, on the other hand, who concentrate on the consciousness of people, describe it as a distorting mask that hides reality.

Each of these perspectives on consciousness has validity. Neuro-scientists are surely correct in saying that consciousness depends on the brain, and therapists are surely right in saying that our thoughts and opinions, because we live with others, can be misdirected. I believe, however, that these professional emphases both distract us from and eclipse what is most crucial about consciousness—that is, what it brings to life.

I have developed my knowledge here—as do almost all doctors who are interested in mental diseases—by noting what patients lose when diseases, such as Alzheimer's, deprive them of full conscious-ness. As a result I've become less concerned about how consciousness is generated, which is an issue that can preoccupy neuroscientists, or about how consciousness can go awry, an issue that can preoccupy therapists. I stress what consciousness is and what it means for humankind—its implications rather than its subordinations.

Consciousness is a phenomenon of nature. As such, it brings an enormous enhancement to the executive power of any creature that has it, a capability demonstrated by the achievements of the scientists themselves employing their consciousness. In fact, an evolutionary view reveals that the emergence of consciousness released those ani-mals in which it first glimmered from automatic responses to their environment. They could plan with both past experiences and pres-ent goals "in mind" rather than respond reflexively to the stimuli striking them.

To be direct: consciousness introduced freedom into nature by enhancing choice and robust unpredictability—that is, the radical contingency of insight. With the emergence of humankind, this ca-pacity for freedom derived from insightful consciousness became a radical, fundamental, and defining aspect of our being. By the light of consciousness our behaviors emerge as more and more considered, more and more responsible, and less and less determined. Far from a "folkish" mirage or a self-serving mask, consciousness exists to reveal and impel us toward the truth, to liberate us more and more from biological, psychological, and social burdens, and to permit our best intentions to blossom.

This conception, although acknowledging the viewpoints of the two groups with whom I work, moves beyond them. By emphasizing what "is" in human nature, namely, a consciousness capable of progressing toward truth, this conception immediately imposes an "ought" upon our relationships with each other. Specifically, this concept encourages us to build a society based on justice, consciously appreciated, coherently explained, and relentlessly pursued through our capacity to reflect—in mind—on what we have done and what we mean to do.

In the next several decades we shall transcend both the materialism constraining contemporary science and the skepticism impeding the social disciplines by emphasizing the potential for freedom and progress wrapped in human consciousness. We shall underscore, now in the light of better science and humane clinical practice, those convictions employed by such individuals as Ignatius Loyola to build his religious order from which this college takes inspiration and Abraham Lincoln to preserve our country and bring an end to chattel slavery. Human beings, by nature, are free and thus carry—biologically—the contingent possibilities freedom brings. They can be rational, creative, and brave because, through consciousness, they can see the implications of their actions. In words taken from Saint John's Gospel and inscribed in the seal of the Johns Hopkins University whence I come: you shall *know* the truth, and the truth shall make you free. Surely this fact—that our consciousness can know the truth—is worth revisiting again and again, as it gives us confidence in ourselves and each other. Carry that confident opinion from this place in all the enterprises you take on. With it you will achieve mightily and make this world still better. Godspeed.

Another Psychiatrist's Shakespeare

When psychiatrists speak about Shakespeare, as they have done rather often, they usually attend to one of two subjects: the Hamlet problem—what mental hang-up delayed Hamlet's revenge; or the Shakespeare problem—what psychological problems led him to the fantasies of the sonnets or to conflict-driven figures like Othello and Hamlet. Recently I have felt—it may be an occupational hazard—an interest in describing what I see in these works, but I promise to look at the plays just as written to see and evaluate what is obvious there. Their psychological realism should interest psychiatrists and through them others who would mine the works for inspiration. Surely mapping Shakespeare's conscious products (rather than interpreting his unconscious intentions) is a better way to meet him than studying him as though he were a patient who needs to learn what he is "really" thinking.

I shall restrict myself to but a few of Shakespeare's plays and to how Shakespeare approaches mental disorder. But first, I have never been persuaded by the psychoanalytic interpretations of Hamlet from Sigmund Freud and Ernest Jones and dramatically portrayed in Laurence Olivier's movie. For them Hamlet cannot act against his Uncle Claudius because Uncle has done what Hamlet, with his Oedipal conflicts, so wanted to do—kill father and bed mother. I shall return to this conception to place it within what I imagine Shakespeare, the realist, might say about it.

For within all four great tragedies (*Macbeth, Hamlet, King Lear,* and *Othello*), Shakespeare depicts mental disorders vividly. Ophelia, Lear, and Lady Macbeth are all at one time or another severely disturbed, and Shakespeare describes them in ways a psychiatrist can recognize today. As well, other protagonists in the play discuss other forms of psychological unrest such as epilepsy for Macbeth, melancholia for Hamlet, dementia for Lear, and hypersexuality for Desdemona. For all that the placements are in exotic palaces and that these plays were all written within five years of each other, 1601–6, four hundred years ago, the author thinks about the causes of these disorders in a remarkably contemporary way.

He never proposes demonic possession. Although he describes ghosts and witches, he depicts them working on human suspicions and fantasies. He never gives their fell powers control of physical life and existence.

Doctors appear on stage in two of the four plays (*Macbeth* and *Lear*) and act like doctors of today. When Lady Macbeth loses control, walks in her sleep, and reveals her misery and her guilty memories in her talk, her staff calls a doctor (specifically described as a "Doctor of Physic") to observe her.

Shakespeare renders the doctor well. At first, in his authority he gets at the maidservant for bothering him with what might be her own worries. "I have two nights watch'd with you but can perceive no truth in your report. When was it she last walked?" (act 5, scene 1, lines 1–3)—like the resident rounding on the intern: "I don't see your point." But then when Lady Macbeth walks out from her bedroom into the antechamber where the doctor and the servant wait, the doctor goes into action. He takes notes! "I will set down what comes from her, to satisfy my remembrance the more strongly" (5.1.36–38).

That's the familiar fellow. You almost expect him to add (as one might today): "and to satisfy the auditors that I did examine her."

She reveals her guilty secrets in a kind of confused mixture of frightened thoughts and visions. "Out out damned spot! Out I say. What will these hands ne'er be clean?" (5.1.39, 48).

On hearing this, the doctor says directly, "This disease is beyond my practice" (5.1.65), but he later gives it a psychological explanation akin to post-traumatic stress disorder.

> Unnatural deeds do breed unnatural troubles.
> Infected minds to their deaf pillows will discharge their secrets.
> More needs she the divine than the physician. (5.1.79–83)

He does not call for an exorcism of some devil but tells the nurse, "Look after her; Remove from her the means of all annoyance, And still keep eyes upon her" (5.1.83–85). He recognizes both her psychological plight and the danger of suicide, as would a good physician today.

In the next scene, Macbeth himself speaks to the doctor, much as any relative might: "How does your patient, Doctor?" And gets the response:

> Not so sick my lord
> As she is troubled with thick-coming fancies
> That keep her from her rest.

And then Macbeth commands:

> Cure her of that.
> Canst thou not minister to a mind diseas'd,
> Pluck from the memory a rooted sorrow,
> Raze out the written troubles of the brain,
> And with some sweet oblivious antidote
> Cleanse the stuff'd bosom of that perilous stuff
> Which weighs upon the heart?

Again the doctor, given that he recognizes a psychological rather than a physical disorder and sees no place for medication, replies:

> Therein the patient
> Must minister to himself.   (5.2.37–46)

Again Macbeth, not listening to an unwelcome idea and distracted as he prepares for battle, commands the doctor and offers a reward:

> If thou couldst, doctor, cast
> The water of my land, find her disease,
> And purge it to a sound and pristine health,
> I would applaud thee to the very echo,
> That should applaud again.   (5.2.50–54)

He marches off to fight, leaving the doctor deep within the castle mumbling to himself:

> Were I from Dunsinane away and clear,
> Profit again should hardly draw me here.   (5.2.61–62)

Diagnosis, differentiation, prognosis, treatment, and explanation—the ingredients of all doctors' practices are here to see, plus the irritation of trying to help VIPs.

The doctor in *King Lear* is treated better. Lear is delirious and discovered so by his faithful daughter Cordelia, who, calling the doctor, describes Lear to him:

> Alack 'tis he! Why, he was met even now
> As mad, as the vex'd sea, singing aloud,
> Crown'd with rank fumiter and furrow-weeds. (4.4.1–3)

And she asks the doctor:

> What can man's wisdom
> In the restoring his bereaved sense?
> He that helps him take all my outward worth.

The doctor responds:

> There is means, Madam.
> Our foster-nurse of nature is repose,
> The which he lacks; that to provoke in him
> Are many simples operative, whose power
> Will close the eye of anguish. (4.4.8–15)

These medications the doctor provides as we might treat the delirious today. A symptomatic treatment encourages a sleep whence in a subsequent scene Lear awakes, and the doctor's assistants help him through convalescence. On meeting Cordelia now after their bitter quarrel and painful separation, the recovering and repentant Lear can only beg her:

> Pray do not mock me.
> I am a very foolish, fond old man,
> Fourscore and upward, not an hour more nor less
> And, to deal plainly,
> I fear I am not in my perfect mind.

The doctor says then to Cordelia:

> Be comforted, good madam; the great rage,
> You see, is killed in him: and yet it is danger
> to make him even o'er the time he has lost.
> Desire him to go in; trouble him no more till
> further settling. (4.7.59–63, 78–82)

So it is that Shakespeare depicts doctoring and its appropriate status in the care of mental illness. Disruptions of mind and behavior are natural, not supernatural, accessible to our understanding and to natural treatments.

This idea is built on a legacy that goes back to Hippocrates, a legacy not of the completely successful explanations of mental illness—the four humors are no more an accurate explanation than is demonic possession—but of the disease concept, whereby mental symptoms emerge from disruption of the body and brain, an idea that provides confidence that tangible causes do exist, can be found sometime, and when found will determine treatment.

But look—"Not so sick my lord [a]s she is troubled." Psychiatrists accept responsibility for troubles as well as disease, and we appreciate other troubles besides diseases in the protagonists of these tragedies. Indeed all four—Macbeth, Hamlet, Lear, and Othello—are troubled. How does Shakespeare see the genesis of troubles like theirs, and how close would his analysis be to those of today's psychiatrists?

Here again, Shakespeare shuns the primitive claim that these people are "possessed by demons." He is also not tempted by psychic determinism, in which choice, responsibility, redemption, and self-knowledge are illusions, rationalizations in the face of the forces of sexuality, of the economy, of power, or any other supposed fixity of human nature. That these tragic protagonists can misdirect their lives and set in motion forces that destroy them is obvious to Shakespeare, as it should be to us.

In *King Lear* and *Hamlet* Shakespeare turns to temperament—natural distinctions in emotional and behavioral responsiveness that render individuals differently vulnerable to circumstances and different in the way they react to encounters. Shakespeare in *Hamlet* and again in *King Lear* strives to show that in the world actions produce consequences. Not exactly tit for tat, but in a way that we all must notice.

Intellect and temperament influence but do not force the action. Hence the tragedy—the protagonists have the opportunity to avoid their destruction, but each surrenders to his natural bent, and the unintended and unhappy consequences emerge.

Shakespeare in *Hamlet* and in *King Lear* describes the two most familiar polar opposite temperaments: the introvert and the extravert. These temperaments identify not sociability, theatricality, friendliness, as is commonly thought, but rather a characteristic mode of emotional responsiveness.

Extraverts are those with quick emotional responses focused on the moment. This gives them their seeming "warmth" but also their choleric quality. Extraverts can be the life of the party, but, especially with a bit of drink disinhibiting them, they can also become morose and touchy and will sometimes strike out. Lear's tendency to respond to the "moment" generates the action in *King Lear*.

Lear decides—seemingly without much thought—that he will divide his kingdom among his three daughters and then flies into a rage when his favorite, Cordelia, refuses to flatter him so as to receive her portion.

Lear: So young and so untender
Cordelia: So young, my Lord, and true.

Then gets the extravert's outburst:

Lear: Thy truth then be thy dower.   (1.1.108–10)

And when the Earl of Kent, his counselor, tries to intervene to calm him down and make him think about his action, Lear, like some quarrelsome drunk in a tavern, turns on him:

Peace, Kent!
Come not between the dragon and his wrath.   (1.1.123–24)

And drives Kent with Cordelia from the kingdom.

The play devolves from this foolish decision of Lear's and his reactions to those who do not go along with his whims. Shakespeare impresses on the audience that the tendency to precipitate anger and harsh words is a persistent trait of Lear's and these first acts are not just due to an unfortunate momentary lapse. He quarrels later with Goneril, who, for all her evil plans, at this point is merely asking him to quiet his riotous and insolent retinue of servants and knights. She gets in reply:

Lear: Darkness and devils!
              Saddle my horses; call my train together!
              Degenerate bastard! I'll not trouble thee;
              Yet have I left a daughter.   (1.4.273–76)

And certainly the most vicious curse that any parent ever called down upon a child:

Lear: Hear, Nature! Hear, dear goddess, hear:
              Suspend thy purpose, if thou didst intend
              to make this creature fruitful!

Into her womb convey sterility!
Dry up in her the organs of increase,
And from her derogate body never spring
A babe to honor her! If she must teem,
Create her child of spleen, that it may live
And be a thwart disnatured torment to her!
Let it stamp wrinkles in her brow of youth,
With cadent tears fret channels in her cheeks,
Turn all her mother's pains and benefits
To laughter and contempt that she may feel
How sharper than a serpent's tooth it is
To have a thankless child!   (1.4.297–311)

Here Shakespeare depicts an extravert unbridled, unthinking in his responses and unconcerned about their ugly effect on others or the future. The consequences of these acts lead to destruction and to death for both the innocent and the guilty.

Later in the course of the play comes Lear's delirium, but Shakespeare makes his illness one of the consequences, not one of the causes of the action. Tragedy arises from being enwrapped in a temperament and giving way to its promptings even when one senses its impositions.

Lear, like many choleric extraverts, does recognize his folly. He tolerates the fool who accompanies him even when the fool taunts him with what he has done. And because of this insight and the awful pain that comes from recognizing his responsibilities for the sufferings he has brought others, we can pity Lear and partly forgive him at the drama's end. His capacity for repentance and his belated and ultimately fruitless actions to repay all he has injured distinguish the flow of reflective character. With character, the capacity for reform exists, but such reform requires the purging fires of penitential punishment and regret.

The introvert reveals an opposite disposition. His or her emotional response is slow to grow but builds in intensity over time. It may be long unexpressed and dissipates only slowly. The attention of the introvert is drawn by the implications of encounters and the likely future they portend. As the vivid emotional expression of the extravert is choler, that of the introvert is melancholy. Lear is the prototypic choleric extravert, Hamlet the prototypic melancholic introvert.

The play starts with Hamlet grieving over his father's sudden death, and, humiliated by the disclosure of his mother's emotional shallowness and coarse sensuality, he falls into a state of deep and abiding melancholy sapping his power of action while encouraging habits of reflection.

Hamlet: O God! God!
How weary, stale, flat, and unprofitable,
Seems to me all the uses of this world!
Fie on't! Oh fie, fie! 'Tis an unweeded garden,
That grows to seed; things rank and gross in nature
Possess it merely.   (1.2.132–35)

He is prone to self-lacerating feelings that further render him impotent to be either at the royal court or at his university.

And just then, as we grasp this disposition of his through and through, comes the encounter with the ghost of his dead father, who confirms some of Hamlet's inchoate suspicions by describing his mother's adultery and his own murder at his brother Claudius's hand. The ghost demands that Hamlet "revenge his foul and most unnatural murder" (1.5.25).

The implication is that Hamlet will act, and he certainly at first responds by asking for more knowledge so that he can respond appropriately:

Haste me to know't, that I, with wings as swift
As meditation or the thoughts of love,
May sweep to my revenge.   (1.5.29–30)

But instead of "sweeping," as would a Lear, he leaves the battlements of Elsinore agonizing:

The time is out of joint;—O cursed spite,
That ever I was born to set it right!   (1.5.189–90)

The introvert's reflections sap his strength, impede action, and produce tragedy. He knows the situation calls for prompt action—some expression of the motto that inspires every great surgeon, "a chance to cut is a chance to cure!" But he waits.

Again, it is not disease that inhibits Hamlet. He is capable of vigorous actions: he kills Polonius with dispatch and shows no regret even as this act destroys Ophelia's mind and launches Laertes on his own mission of revenge. He has a lively wit and, most important, great clarity of thought—both features seen in how he disposes of the two treacherous former school fellows, Rosencrantz and Guildenstern, "whom I will trust as I will adders fanged" (3.4.203). It is rather his slowness in responding to things more crucial to him that renders his actions so deliberate and ineffectual. This feature is at the heart of the play.

As with Lear, Hamlet notices his own emotional character, and it mystifies him. He even points out how one of the players he hired is capable of displaying feelings for a myth and presumes his livelier emotions would prompt the fellow to action.

> Hamlet: What's Hecuba to him or he to Hecuba
> That he should weep for her? What would he do,
> Had he the motive and the cue for passion that I have?
> (2.2.585–88)

This is again the feature of temperament. The subjects identify it. They are in it, indeed sense it, but do not so understand it. Psychiatrists attempt to guide such troubled people and strengthen them in their encounters.

But even psychiatrists might agree there is plenty of reason for Hamlet's hesitation. The message, after all, is delivered by a ghost—a personage who depicts the consequences of death, the losses of "here" and the great mysteries of "there":

> To die; to sleep;—
> To sleep? Perchance to dream! Ay, there's the rub;
> For in that sleep of death what dreams may come,
> When we have shuffl'd off this mortal coil,
> Must give us pause. (3.1.64–68)

And surely here is where Freud and Jones come in—how their idea cuts through this "surface" description of temperament and proposes a deeper meaning to Hamlet's demoralization and ineptitude. He is not paralyzed and self-mystified because his introvert's disposition renders him melancholic and demoralized. He cannot act because secretly, unconsciously, he identifies with his uncle, who accomplished what Hamlet himself desired. Of course, no evidence for these desires emerges in the play, and none can be found even within the sources of Shakepeare's tale. So it's an explanation of Hamlet's hesitation that depends for its proof on Hamlet's hesitation—a circular reasoning that emerges too often in psychiatric discourse. Perhaps, though, one can claim that Hamlet protests *too* much about his mother's sensuality, or perhaps one could draw the claim from Hamlet's going to her bedroom to persuade her to alter her behavior. But fundamentally the only evidence is his failure to act against Claudius, and that cannot be used to prove what the unconscious motive was purporting to explain.

However, it remains a powerful—and has been to many a persuasive—explanation because it tells another story from within the play and seems to grasp Hamlet's psychological unrest at several levels of analysis simultaneously. Not only the action and its consequences but also his hesitation, his self-blame, and even perhaps his temperament itself are explained.

Introversion is seen as the outcome of a kind of repressed guilt over sexual impulses. For such a gain, who wants to quibble over logic? The story speaks beyond professed motives to subterranean springs of energy, to something out of conscious awareness or disposition. It is so wondrously deep, mysterious, and unexpected, it must be true.

And this leads me to my last Shakespearean tragedy and last sense of Shakespeare as a realist and would-be critic of Freud. Shakespeare is not without an appreciation of the power of stories but rather demonstrates that they can provoke actions and cause tragedy. He displays these facts in *Othello,* in which they are employed for many purposes. Stories generate opinions, actions, and consequences without much regard for their truth, falseness, or even logic. In *Othello* Shakespeare demonstrates why stories, of all our ways of knowing and teaching, must be most closely and critically appraised.

For the tragedy of Othello is a play about a man who at first succeeds with a story by which he seduces and persuades and then is undone by another story in which he is tricked and provoked into a blind murderous jealousy. We sit back in amazement of the events as they transpire.

The play opens with a clamor of Brabantio, Desdemona's father, who, learning that the black Othello has married his daughter, presumes that he has worked some magic on her:

Oh thou foul thief, where hast thou stow'd my daughter?
Damned as thou art, thou hast enchanted her;
For I'll refer me to all things of sense,
If she in chains of magic were not bound,
Whether a maid so tender, fair, and happy,
So opposite to marriage that she shunned
The wealthy curled darlings of our nation,
Would ever have, t' incur a general mock,
Run from her guardage to the sooty bosom
Of such a thing as thou—to fear, not to delight.
Judge me the world, if 'tis not gross in sense
That thou has practis'd on her with foul charms,
Abused her delicate youth with drugs or minerals
That weakens motion.   (1.2.62–75)

Accusing Othello of magic or some pharmacologic foul means, Brabantio demands that the Duke of Venice hear him out and punish Othello as some kind of foul wizard or trafficker in illegal drugs and aphrodisiacs. Yet Othello testifies to his taking of Desdemona in a set of remarkable responses.

I will a round, unvarnished tale deliver
Of my whole course of love—what drugs, what charms,
What conjuration, and what mighty magic
(For such proceeding I am charged withal),
I won his daughter.   (1.3.90–94)

And when given the opportunity to defend himself continues:

Her father lov'd me, oft invited me;
Still question'd me the story of my life
From year to year—the battles, sieges, fortunes
That I have pass'd.
I ran it through, even from my boyish days
To th' very moment that he bade me tell it;
Wherein I spoke of most disastrous chances,
Of moving accidents by flood and field,
Of hair-breadth scapes i' th' imminent deadly breach,
Of being taken by the insolent foe
And sold to slavery, of my redemption thence
And portance in my travel's history;

Wherein of antres vast and deserts idle,
Rough quarries, rocks, and hills whose heads touch heaven,
It was my hint to speak—such was my process,—
And of the Cannibals that each other eat,
The Anthropophagi, and men whose heads
Do grow beneath their shoulders. These to hear
Would Desdemona seriously incline;
But still the house affairs would draw her thence,
Which ever as she could with haste dispatch,
She'd come again, and with a greedy ear
Devour up my discourse: Which I observing,
Took once a pliant hour, and found good means
To draw from her a prayer of earnest heart
That I would all my pilgrimage dilate,
Whereof by parcels she had something heard,
But not intentively. I did consent,
And often did beguile her of her tears,
When I did speak of some distressful stroke
That my youth suffer'd. My story being done,
She gave me for my pains a world of sighs;
She swore, in faith 'twas strange, 'twas passing strange,
'Twas pitiful, 'twas wondrous pitiful.
She'd wish'd she had not heard it; yet she wish'd
That heaven had made her such a man. She thank'd me,
And bade me, if I had a friend that lov'd her,
I should but teach him how to tell my story.
And that would woo her. Upon this hint I spake:
She lov'd me for the dangers I had pass'd,
And I lov'd her that she did pity them.
This only is the witchcraft I have us'd.   (1.3.128–69)

And to this the listening and judging Duke responds: "I think this tale would win my daughter too" (1.3.171).

Othello wins Desdemona's love through his telling of a story full of excitement, meaning, and tragedy. But "This only is the witchcraft I have us'd" is a telling *only* because the rest of the play depicts the collapse of this soldier, his encasement in jealous passion and anger *only* by another story. Again—no drugs, no witchcraft—told to him by Iago, the villain, who for no other reason than malice itself can get

Othello entangled in the belief that Desdemona has loved Cassio and still enjoys his favors, speaks for him, and hides her love from Othello. So says Iago:

> The Moor is of a free and open nature,
> That thinks men honest that but seem to be so,
> And will tenderly be led by the nose
> As asses are.
> I have it. It is engendered. Hell and night
> Must bring this monstrous birth to light.   (1.3.405–10)

Once persuaded by Iago's story, then, without the simplest checking for solid evidence from other informants, Othello is overmastered and kills Desdemona despite her pitiful protests—in fact discounting all that she says and refusing to let her bring testimony in defense. When Othello enters the bedroom to strangle Desdemona, his first words reveal his commitment to a cause-and-effect view of the situation:

> It is the cause, it is the cause, my soul,—
> Let me not name it to you, you chaste stars!
> It is the cause. Yet I'll not shed her blood,
> Nor scar that whiter skin of hers than snow,
> And smooth as monumental alabaster.
> Yet she must die, else she'll betray more men.
> Put out the light, and then put out the light.   (5.2.1–7)

But there is no "cause" for action because, as Othello will soon learn, Desdemona's adultery and supposed hypersexuality are all story-driven illusions by which Iago has gulled him. The story and the events it proposes seem a way to knowledge but prove a way to mischief. This is the heart of *Othello*. We might think of its message when we are told a story about Hamlet's behavior. And wonder whether we are better for its purported sense of him or whether it in a sense murders the meaning and debases the tragic vision of that play.

In *Othello*, Shakespeare, in the most ingenious way, shows us the dangers of the story. Stories often appear to be a source of information when in fact they aim to persuade—and in Othello and Desdemona's situation, to court and seduce.

A story can intend to change the way we look at a situation and to set a new idea in motion. It can enlarge our understanding and our aims, but it may raise awkward, spoiling, cynical, sour questions. It may be a duplicitous manipulation. This is, I think, the best answer to the Freudian interpretation of Hamlet and would, I believe, be given by Shakespeare himself if he were asked. Beware the story; its power is outside facts and may simply, even as it uses facts, play upon your suspicions and mislead. What looks like depth may well be distortion and deceit.

Shakespeare is our contemporary. He deals with so much and even shows us psychiatrists how we might function with understanding.

In his realism Shakespeare offers not an "essence" of humankind, a single vision of our minds, but a multiplicity of visions, each of which carries a message for reflections. The Shakespeare of these tragedies is certain of three things: evil people exist, many of the best people are flawed, and actions generated by evil ideas inadequately confronted will bring about an appalling and brutal justice whereby both the guilty and the innocent suffer. Was there truer reality for us, who live in a time of pestilence and terror, to contemplate?

Surgical Sex

When the practice of sex-change surgery first emerged back in the early 1970s, I would often remind its advocating psychiatrists that with other patients, alcoholics in particular, they would quote the Serenity Prayer, "God, give me the serenity to accept the things I cannot change, the courage to change the things I can, and the wisdom to know the difference." Where did they get the idea that our sexual identity (*gender* was the term they preferred) as men or women was in the category of things that could be changed?

Their regular response was to show me their patients. Men (and until recently they were all men) with whom I spoke before their surgery would tell me that their bodies and sexual identities were at variance. Those I met after surgery would tell me that the surgery and hormone treatments that had made them "women" had also made them happy and contented. None of these encounters were persuasive, however. The postsurgical subjects struck me as caricatures of women. They wore high heels, copious makeup, and flamboyant clothing; they spoke about how they found themselves able to give vent to their natural inclinations for peace, domesticity, and gentleness—but their large hands, prominent Adam's apples, and thick facial features were incongruous (and would become more so as they aged). Female psychiatrists whom I sent to talk with them would intuitively see through the disguise and the exaggerated postures. "Gals know gals," one said to me, "and that's a guy."

The subjects before the surgery struck me as even stranger as they struggled to convince anyone who might influence the decision for their surgery. First, they spent an unusual amount of time thinking and talking about sex and their sexual experiences; their sexual hungers and adventures seemed to preoccupy them. Second, discussion of babies or children provoked little interest from them; indeed, they seemed indifferent to children. But third, and most remarkable, many of these men-who-claimed-to-be-women reported that they found women sexually attractive and that they saw themselves as "lesbians." When I noted to their champions that their psychological leanings seemed more like those of men than of women, I would get various replies, mostly to the effect that in making such judgments I was drawing on sexual stereotypes.

Until 1975, when I became psychiatrist-in-chief at the Johns Hopkins Hospital, I could usually keep my own counsel on these matters. But once I was given authority over all the practices in the Psychiatry Department, I realized that if I remained passive, I would be tacitly co-opted in encouraging sex-change surgery in the very department that had originally proposed and still defended it. I decided to challenge what I considered to be a misdirection of psychiatry and to demand more information both before and after their operations.

Two issues presented themselves as targets for study. First, I wanted to test the claim that men who had undergone sex-change surgery found resolution for their many general psychological problems. Second (and this was more ambitious), I wanted to see whether male infants with ambiguous genitalia who were being surgically transformed into females and raised as girls did, as the theory (again from Hopkins) claimed, settle easily into the sexual identity that was chosen for them. These claims had generated the opinion in psychiatric circles that one's "sex" and one's "gender" were distinct matters, sex being genetically and hormonally determined from conception, while gender was culturally shaped by the actions of family and others during childhood.

The first issue was easier and required only that I encourage the ongoing research of a member of the faculty who was an accomplished student of human sexual behavior. The psychiatrist and psychoanalyst Jon Meyer was already developing a means of following up with adults who received sex-change operations at Hopkins in order to see how much the surgery had helped them. He found that most of the patients he tracked down some years after their surgery were contented with what they had done and that only a few regretted it. But in every other respect, they were little changed in their psychological condition. They had much the same problems with relationships, work, and emotions as before. The hope that they would emerge now from their emotional difficulties to flourish psychologically had not been fulfilled.

We saw the results as demonstrating that just as these men enjoyed cross-dressing as women before the operation so they enjoyed cross-living after it. But they were no better in their psychological integration or any easier to live with. With these facts in hand I concluded that Hopkins was fundamentally cooperating with a mental illness. We psychiatrists, I thought, would do better to concentrate on trying to fix their minds and not their genitalia.

Thanks to this research, Dr. Meyer was able to make some sense of the mental disorders that were driving this request for unusual and radical treatment. Most of the cases fell into one of two quite different groups. One group consisted of conflicted and guilt-ridden homosexual men who saw a sex change as a way to resolve their conflicts over homosexuality by allowing them to behave sexually as females with men. The other group, mostly older men, consisted of heterosexual (and some bisexual) males who found intense sexual arousal in cross-dressing as females. As they had grown older, they had become eager to add more verisimilitude to their costumes and either sought or had suggested to them a surgical transformation that would include breast implants, penile amputation, and pelvic reconstruction to resemble a woman.

Further study of similar subjects in the psychiatric services of the Clark Institute in Toronto identified these men by the autoarousal they experienced in imitating sexually seductive females. Many of them imagined that their displays might be sexually arousing to onlookers, especially to females. This idea, a form of "sex in the head" (D. H. Lawrence), was what provoked their first adventure in dressing up in women's undergarments and had eventually led them toward the surgical option. Because most of them found women to be the objects of their interest, they identified themselves to the psychiatrists as lesbians. The name eventually coined in Toronto to describe this form of sexual misdirection was "autogynephilia." Once again I concluded that to provide a surgical alteration to the body of these unfortunate people was to collaborate with a mental disorder rather than to treat it.

This information and the improved understanding of what we had been doing led us to stop prescribing sex-change operations for adults at Hopkins—much, I'm glad to say, to the relief of several of our plastic surgeons who had previously been commandeered to carry out the procedures. And with this solution to the first issue I could turn to the second—namely, the practice of surgically assigning femaleness to male newborns who at birth had malformed, sexually ambiguous genitalia and severe phallic defects. This practice, more the province of the Pediatric Department than of my own, was nonetheless of concern to psychiatrists because the opinions generated around these cases helped to form the view that sexual identity was a matter of cultural conditioning rather than something fundamental to the human constitution.

Several conditions, fortunately rare, can lead to the misconstruction of the genitourinary tract during embryonic life. When such a condition occurs in a male, the easiest form of plastic surgery by far, with a view to correcting the abnormality and gaining a cosmetically satisfactory appearance, is to remove all the male parts, including the testes, and to construct from the tissues available a labial and vaginal configuration. This action provides these malformed babies with female-looking genital anatomy regardless of their genetic sex. Given the claim that the sexual identity of the child would easily follow the genital appearance if backed up by familial and cultural support, the pediatric surgeons took to constructing female-like genitalia for both females with an XX chromosome constitution and males with an XY so as to make them all look like little girls, and they were to be raised as girls by their parents.

All this was done, of course, with the consent of the parents, who, distressed by these grievous malformations in their newborns, were persuaded by the pediatric endocrinologists and consulting psychologists to accept transformational surgery for their sons. They were told that their child's sexual identity (again his "gender") would simply conform to environmental conditioning. If the parents consistently responded to the child as a girl now that his genital structure resembled a girl's, he would accept that role without much travail.

This proposal presented the parents with a critical decision. The doctors increased the pressure behind the proposal by noting to the parents that a decision had to be made promptly because a child's sexual identity settles in by about age two or three. The process of inducing the child into the female role should start immediately, with name, birth certificate, baby paraphernalia, and so on. With the surgeons ready and the physicians confident, the parents were faced with an offer difficult to refuse (although, interestingly, a few parents did refuse this advice and decided to let nature take its course).

I thought these professional opinions and the choices being pressed on the parents rested upon anecdotal evidence that was hard to verify and even harder to replicate. Despite the confidence of their advocates, they lacked substantial empirical support. I encouraged one of our resident psychiatrists, William G. Reiner (already interested in the subject because prior to his psychiatric training he had been a pediatric urologist and had witnessed the problem from the other side), to set about doing a systematic follow-up of these children—particularly the males transformed into females in infancy—so as to determine just how sexually integrated they became as adults.

The results here were even more startling than in Meyer's work. Reiner picked out for intensive study cloacal exstrophy because it would best test the idea that cultural influence plays the foremost role in producing sexual identity. Cloacal exstrophy is an embryonic misdirection that produces a gross abnormality of pelvic anatomy such that the bladder and the genitalia are badly deformed at birth. The male penis fails to form, and the bladder and urinary tract are not separated distinctly from the gastrointestinal tract. But crucial to Reiner's study is the fact that the embryonic development of these unfortunate males is not hormonally different from that of normal males. They develop within a male-typical prenatal hormonal milieu provided by their Y chromosome and by their normal testicular function. This exposes these growing embryos/fetuses to the male hormone testosterone—just like all males in their mother's womb.

Although animal research had long since shown that male sexual behavior is directly derived from this exposure to testosterone during embryonic life, this fact did not deter the pediatric practice of surgically treating male infants with this grievous anomaly by castration (amputating their testes and any vestigial male genital structures) and vaginal construction so that they could be raised as girls. This practice had become almost universal by the mid-1970s. Such cases offered Reiner the best test of the two aspects of the doctrine underlying such treatment: (1) that humans at birth are neutral as to their sexual identity, and (2) that for humans it is the postnatal, cultural, nonhormonal influences, especially those of early childhood, that most influence their ultimate sexual identity. Males with cloacal exstrophy were regularly altered surgically to resemble females, and their parents were instructed to raise them as girls. But would the fact that they had had the full testosterone exposure in utero defeat the attempt to raise them as girls? Answers might become evident with the careful follow-up that Reiner was launching.

Before describing his results, I should note that the doctors proposing this treatment for the males with cloacal exstrophy understood and acknowledged that they were introducing a number of new and severe physical problems for these males. These infants, of course, had no ovaries, and their testes were surgically amputated, which meant that they had to receive exogenous hormones for life. They would also be denied by the same surgery any opportunity for fertility later on. One could not ask the little patient about his willingness to pay this price. These were considered by the physicians advising the parents to be acceptable burdens to bear in order to avoid distress in childhood about malformed genital structures, and it was hoped that they could follow a conflict-free direction in their maturation as girls and women.

Reiner, however, discovered that such reengineered males were almost never comfortable as females once they became aware of themselves and the world. From the start of their active play life, they behaved spontaneously like boys and were obviously different from their sisters and other girls, enjoying rough-and-tumble games but not dolls and "playing house." Later on, most of those individuals who learned that they were actually genetic males wanted to reconstitute their lives as males (some even asked for surgical reconstruction and male hormone replacement)—and all this despite the earnest efforts by their parents to treat them as girls.

Reiner's results, reported in the January 22, 2004, issue of the *New England Journal of Medicine,* are worth recounting. He followed up sixteen genetic males with cloacal exstrophy seen at Hopkins, of whom fourteen underwent neonatal assignment to femaleness socially, legally, and surgically. The other two parents refused the advice of the pediatricians and raised their sons as boys. Eight of the fourteen subjects assigned to be females had since declared themselves to be male. Five were living as females, and one lived with unclear sexual identity. The two raised as males had remained male. All sixteen of these people had interests that were typical of males, such as hunting, ice hockey, karate, and bobsledding. Reiner concluded from this work that the sexual identity followed the genetic constitution. Male-type tendencies (vigorous play, sexual arousal by females, and physical aggressiveness) followed the testosterone-rich intrauterine fetal development of the people he studied, regardless of efforts to socialize them as females after birth.

Having looked at the Reiner and Meyer studies, we in the Johns Hopkins Psychiatry Department eventually concluded that human sexual identity is mostly built into our constitution by the genes we inherit and the embryogenesis we undergo. Male hormones sexualize the brain and the mind. Sexual dysphoria—a sense of disquiet in one's sexual role—naturally occurs among those rare males who are raised as females in an effort to correct an infantile genital structural problem. A seemingly similar disquiet can be socially induced in apparently constitutionally normal males, in association with (and presumably prompted by) serious behavioral aberrations, among which are conflicted homosexual orientations and the remarkable male deviation now called autogynephilia.

Quite clearly, then, we psychiatrists should work to discourage those adults who seek surgical sex reassignment. When Hopkins announced that it would stop doing these procedures in adults with sexual dysphoria, many other hospitals followed suit, but some medical centers still carry out this surgery. Thailand has several centers that do the surgery "no questions asked" for anyone with the money to pay for it and the means to travel to Thailand. I am disappointed but not surprised by this, given that some surgeons and medical centers can be persuaded to carry out almost any kind of surgery when pressed by patients with sexual deviations, especially if those patients find a psychiatrist to vouch for them. The most astonishing example is the surgeon in England who is prepared to amputate the legs of patients who claim to find sexual excitement in gazing at and exhibiting stumps of amputated legs. At any rate, we at Hopkins hold that official psychiatry has good evidence to argue against this kind of treatment and should begin to close down the practice everywhere.

For children with birth defects the most rational approach at this moment is to correct promptly any of the major urological defects they face but to postpone any decision about sexual identity until much later, while raising the child according to its genetic sex. Medical caretakers and parents can strive to make the child aware that aspects of sexual identity will emerge as he or she grows. Settling on what to do about it should await maturation and the child's appreciation of his or her own identity.

Proper care, including good parenting, means helping the child through the medical and social difficulties presented by the genital anatomy but in the process protecting what tissues can be retained, in particular the gonads. This effort must continue to the point where the child can see the problem of a life role more clearly as a sexually differentiated individual emerges from within. Then as the young person gains a sense of responsibility for the result, he or she can be helped through any surgical constructions that are desired. Genuine informed consent derives only from the person who is going to live with the outcome and cannot rest upon the decisions of others who believe they "know best."

How are these ideas now being received? I think tolerably well. The "transgender" activists (now often allied with gay liberation movements) still argue that their members are entitled to whatever surgery they want, and they still claim that their sexual dysphoria represents a true conception of their sexual identity. They have made some protests against the diagnosis of autogynephilia as a mechanism to generate demands for sex-change operations, but they have offered little evidence to refute the diagnosis. Psychiatrists are taking better sexual histories from those requesting sex-change surgery and are discovering more examples of this strange male exhibitionist proclivity.

Much of the enthusiasm for the quick-fix approach to birth defects expired when the anecdotal evidence about the much publicized case of a male twin raised as a girl proved to be bogus. The psychologist in charge hid, by actually misreporting, the news that the boy, despite the efforts of his parents to treat him and raise him as a girl, had constantly challenged their treatment of him, ultimately found out about the deception, and restored himself as a male. Sadly, he carried an additional diagnosis of major depression and ultimately committed suicide.

I think the issue of sex change for males is no longer one in which much can be said for the other side. But I have learned from the experience that the toughest challenge is trying to gain agreement to seek empirical evidence for opinions about sex and sexual behavior, even when the opinions seem on their face unreasonable. One might expect that those who claim that sexual identity has no biological or physical basis would bring forth more evidence to persuade others. But as I've learned, there is a deep prejudice in favor of the idea that nature is totally malleable.

Without any fixed position on what is given in human nature, any manipulation of it can be defended as legitimate. A practice that appears to give people what they want—and what some of them are prepared to clamor for—turns out to be difficult to combat with ordinary professional experience and wisdom. Even controlled trials or careful follow-up studies to ensure that the practice itself is not damaging are often resisted and the results rejected.

I have witnessed a great deal of damage from sex reassignment. The children transformed from their male constitution into female roles suffered prolonged distress and misery as they sensed their natural attitudes. Their parents usually lived with guilt over their decisions—second-guessing themselves and somewhat ashamed of the fabrication, both surgical and social, they have imposed on their sons. As for the adults who came to us claiming to have discovered their "true" sexual identity and to have heard about sex-change operations, we psychiatrists have been distracted from studying the causes and natures of their mental misdirections by preparing them for surgery and for a life in the other sex. We have wasted scientific and technical resources and damaged our professional credibility by collaborating with madness rather than trying to study, cure, and ultimately prevent it.

First Things, 2004

No Veterinarian to "The Naked Ape"

As I recount to colleagues our debate within the President's Council on Bioethics leading to the publication of the book *Beyond Therapy: Biotechnology and the Pursuit of Happiness* (2003), many ask, "Why are you guys worrying about the off-label use of medications" such as growth hormones, steroids, stimulants, and antidepressants? By "off-label" they mean the use of these drugs and hormones not, as originally intended, to cure people of conditions such as depression, infection, or hormone deficiency but to enable the healthy to become stronger, quicker, or taller than they would be naturally. "After all," they note, "who's to say where sickness ends and health begins—and anyway, why can't folks try stuff as long as it doesn't hurt them?"

These natural questions are relatively easy to answer, as they all in some way turn on concerns over the risks involved in taking medications. But I remind my interlocutors that people do certainly sense other problems in "off-label" medications and express their concerns. Witness the recent outcry in the newspapers, picked up and amplified by the president's State of the Union address, over major league baseball players who increased their strength—and disrupted the credibility of their records—by using muscle-enhancing steroids and growth hormones on the advice of their trainers and physicians.

Some critics of this practice were concerned over the risks to health these professional athletes were prepared (or pressured) to accept. Indeed, these risks are not trivial. But many more were troubled by what biologic enhancements implied about the meaning of achievement in sports and the values expressed in athletic competition.

A Question of Purpose

Several of my questioners did identify this challenging question from the controversy over sports by asking: "Just what are you trying to preserve or defend when you debate the use of medications to enhance some trait, rather than treat an illness?" I hold that answering this question of purpose is central not only to the sports issue but also to the mission of the council itself. Therefore, I begin by noting how this council was charged by the president to spur public discussion on bioethics in a fashion that would get beyond some simple calculus of risks and benefits to consider what challenges to human values and moral purpose the new discoveries in biomedicine could bring to us as people. Sports are one arena in which such challenges would emerge, but hardly the only one.

Specifically, in working with our chairman, Leon Kass, to produce *Beyond Therapy*, we council members explored how medications with effects on mood and cognition, so useful in treating certain mental disorders, might alter a doctor's practice with people seeking to enhance desirable traits.

Doctors, after all, do not see themselves as veterinarians to Desmond Morris's *Naked Ape*—workers who tinker with the bodily structure and function of a human as if they were simply beefing up a biologic machine. They hold that, as advisers and teachers, they treat people who need more than technological know-how in order to thrive, who need help to understand what goes into a good human life and how it can go awry. However, as information spreads about medications, some patients—perhaps better called "clients"—are turning up asking for and expecting novel pharmacologic services from their doctors, services that may not extend the patients' best interests. *Beyond Therapy* intends to spur the public to think about these matters.

Case examples help make these ideas about apt and inapt use of medications—especially the newly discovered medications—clear. Here are three, chosen because each depicts a particular aspect of contemporary life in a psychiatric practice and represents a situation in which human hopes and fears are in play. In each, medications are an issue even though a "quick fix" with some medication not only would have fallen short of a solution but might well have distracted everyone from the central and deeply human issues at the heart of the problem.

A Frustrated Young Man

To begin: at least once a year, I am asked to see some young man (seldom a young woman) whose parents worry about his school performance and are wondering whether some medications—either sedatives for his mild test anxiety or stimulants for his mild distractibility—might enhance it. The parents are gifted professionals with long records of academic success and honors (valedictorians, Phi Beta Kappa election, etc.). They worry that their son's present school record and lack of scholastic achievements matching theirs indicate either that something is wrong with him that I might fix with one of these new medications they have read about or that he has some unapparent psychological conflict that I might resolve for him.

The truth is that the son does not have the superior IQ of his parents. The statistical "reversion to the mean" inherent in the genetic roulette of a polygenic feature such as IQ has brought him a somewhat lower capacity than that of his gifted parents. But often he, and subjects like him, more than balance this aspect of their makeup by displaying—and in fact surpassing their parents in—several other fine human characteristics. He may be handsome, charming, athletic, graceful. These traits are visible and acknowledged by all, even though, on the day I see him, his most prominent feature is his frustration over disappointing his parents.

My task in this situation is to get the parents to forget about adjusting him to their aims with medications or anything else. I want them to appreciate what he brings to them and to all of us in life-affirming ways. I point out that no one can "major in IQ" in life, but anyone can use a whole variety of assets to make life work for him or her. These parents need to understand the young man for what he is and use their talents—and social connections if need be—to guide him toward enterprises that will employ his particular talents and skills to build a life and a career. They should emphasize his strengths, stop trying to make him more like themselves, and give up their notion (common, I've discovered, among the gifted) that the only path to success in life is the one they followed.

I do not immediately succeed in this process with some of these parents, primarily because at the start they assume that my job is to do their bidding and "fix" the young man rather than reinterpret their situation for them. But with time I can usually win them over, thanks mainly to the natural affection all parents have for their offspring but also because I, an outsider, embarrassed them into thinking about the gifts of life by emphasizing what is attractive about their son.

Right Feelings, Wrong Objects

Here is a second prototypic example of how assumptions about life can, in the present era, prompt a search for enhancement medications that misses the point. A young woman arrives in my office depressed and concerned about what she imagines to be some flaw in her psychological makeup that renders her unattractive to others. Her concerns, it turns out, have emerged from several failed romances. Each seems to have followed the same course: she meets an attractive young man and develops a relationship that rather promptly—as is customary with young people now—becomes an intimate one. After some months, and just as she has begun to hope they will marry and start a family together, he tells her he is "not ready" for such a serious commitment and its attendant responsibilities. She concludes he is not sufficiently interested in her, and soon they part.

The repetitiveness of this experience—right down to the stock expression "I'm not ready"—leads her to believe that something about her is to blame. She wonders, as she reflects on her feelings and her behavior, if she's "too intense," "too possessive," or "too needy." She's certainly disheartened and demoralized, and she asks me for medication for her mood and perhaps some other medications that would reduce her anxiety around men—making her perhaps more "relaxed" about these matters.

I notice how she is distressed and concerned about male withdrawal but seeks to explain it as a result of her shortcomings. With these ideas in my mind, I try to show her that, in expecting intimacy to lead to commitment, she is the one who is acting in a natural way, and her boyfriends are not. I tell her that she needs neither a sedative for her thoughts nor an antidepressant to rid her of her low mood but a better assessment of the situation she faces.

When I eventually point out how contemporary sexual mores, supported by easy contraception, tend to emphasize what one receives from an intimate relationship rather than what one brings to it—that is, taking something from one another rather than making something together—she may wonder, primarily because she has never heard such ideas from a doctor, whether she has come to the right office. Only after figuratively catching her breath does she ask exactly what I think she should do in these situations. I respond to this question by saying she will need some coaching or "cognitive-behavioral" psychotherapy as she approaches affectionate relationships in the future. I suggest several therapists—usually female—who have helped other young women I referred.

She came with the belief that her moods and distress represented some set of pathologic features in herself. I try to help her appreciate that she has been cooperating with a cultural system that permits males to remain perpetual adolescents (and even offers them a standard excuse line, "I'm not ready"), postponing indefinitely their transition into responsible—read "stand-up"—men. Her goal should be to figure out how to stop cooperating with this system and its misuse of her.

Tempting Thoughts

As a final example of the temptation to use pharmacologic tools for enhancement I offer an experience and thought experiment from my personal, rather than professional, life. I enjoy periodic, several-day visits from my eight-year-old grandson. We do many things together, but one of our favorite activities is playing chess and analyzing situations on the board. He's pretty good for a youngster, and for a period of about half to three-quarters of an hour, we can concentrate together on these problems.

But as the time passes, I sense his attention waning, and eventually—sooner that I do—he wearies of these "if the opponent makes that move then we should follow with this response" analyses. I've learned to offer him something else to do with me then—best something more physical such as running or throwing a ball—all with the tacit agreement that "maybe later" we could return to chess.

The thought experiment, though, comes as I realize how, with a medication such as Ritalin, I could hold him longer at the chessboard, enjoy the interplay with him for a greater stretch of time, and even, so I might rationalize, make him a better player. The thought is enough to identify the injustice. To use my medical skills to draw something I want from him rather than to accept and support the break from effort his nature seeks is to deny, indeed belittle, his boyhood. "More recess, less Ritalin" I regularly prescribe to people worried about how boys tend to be restless in class. I'm even more confident of the wisdom in that prescription after spending time so happily with a first-rate example of the group.

Cheating Victory of Its Meaning

With these case examples in mind, let us now return to the sports problem that may be the greatest source of public interest and disquiet over pharmacologic enhancements today. I hold that the expressions of concern brought out in those discussions resemble in many ways the concerns raised in my clinical examples. I also believe that some aspects of the solutions likely to be effective for these athletes will apply to practice with patients such as I've described. Much will depend on attitudes in the community about what is to be admired and what is to be scorned, about what advances and what retards our human pursuits.

William James referred to organized sports as "the moral equivalent of war." And for most of us that's just why we are drawn to the games, as both players and spectators. Nowhere else can we see human beings struggling to be their best, displaying the strenuous, dare one say manly, virtues of courage, tenacity, and self-sacrifice for some collective victory in an arena in which blood is not shed and lives are not lost. At their best, organized sports work as a tangible and direct moral educator to us all by identifying people who have honed wonderful physical gifts and who demonstrate how adversity and stress can be overcome through persistence and bravery put into play with a sense of purpose.

Major league baseball should free itself from the misuse of steroids and other drugs not just by appropriate supervision, rules, and stiff fines but as well by ridicule, contempt, and moral reprobation of the offending athletes by their peers and by the supporters of the game. This reproving stance derives from rejecting the "anything goes" view of athletic competitions and is inspired by respect for the opportunity in sports to witness remarkable combinations of human gifts and virtues, played out in a framework of conventions that give those gifts and virtues a stage. Artificially altering the players—distorting their bodies and making them somehow chemically different from the rest of us—debases this opportunity.

Most of us can see these points immediately and appreciate that unnatural procedures, by severing performance from effort, cheat victory of its meaning. In the same way, I try to encourage my patients to see the real goals embedded in their pursuit of happiness. Thus I do not aim to cover over a painful but natural response to life circumstances or tone up some cosmetic flaw. Rather, I seek to help a person find coherence and direction in his or her life so as to resolve some of the difficulties prompting the trip to a psychiatrist. "Man does not live on pharmaceuticals alone," we might say today in updating the Gospels. I apply that lesson repeatedly in my office.

Each person in my case examples needed help to recognize just how, like the use of steroids by baseball players, the pharmacologic interventions he or she wanted would be wrong. Here medicating might not be against some formal rule, but it would in important ways distort the goal of treatment and often turn attention away from the real nature of the situation. In all three cases this goal was to recognize the challenging realities built into human life and how best to meet them. The first case illustrated how one should recognize and honor the diversity of excellence to be found among people, the second how to recognize and honor the natural assumptions of human affection, and the last how to recognize and honor psychological characteristics built into and appropriate for the different stages of human development. To intervene with medications in any of these examples might have helped achieve some narrow aim but would have done so at the price of loss of reverence for the good things that life, outside our command, brings to us and prompts us to fulfill.

The Moral Bottom Line

As anyone who reads *Beyond Therapy* will quickly appreciate, the council was not calling for laws to deal with these issues of "off-label" treatments. We thought and wrote differently here than we would about matters in which life and death—or even physical well-being— are involved. Different members brought different experiences with biologic enhancements to this discussion. All, though, wanted to help the public to appreciate both what great goods these new medicines bring to our treatment of the mentally ill and the many aspects of human life at stake as our knowledge in psychopharmacology expands.

In particular I wanted to emphasize what psychiatric practice taught me about what to behold, identify, and admire in individual lives. I've learned that, when no psychiatric illness disrupts the picture and calls for medical relief with these new medications, these assets usually offset the challenging blemishes that remain for each of us to overcome. People triumph over these milder handicaps when they are helped to make sense of their circumstances, live up to their gifts, and cultivate those strenuous virtues of self-sufficiency, energy, loyalty, and independence of mind that grow with practice over time.

The moral "bottom line" for me, a doctor, in the use of all medications (not just the new ones) is: turn to a medication only after you have thought carefully about the patient's symptoms and complaints and decided these issues represent or express some disruption of brain function or structure in need of medical management. Otherwise, help those who consult you to see what they can do to make better sense of their situations and deal more effectively with them. If this method of assessment is followed, then the new discoveries in pharmacology will work as they were designed and a coherent, effective practice of psychiatry will proceed for the benefit of all.

Cerebrum, 2004

Zygote and "Clonote"

The Ethical Use of Embryonic Stem Cells

Bioethics is a debate without rules about a future dimly appre-hended—a debate that is ever in danger of slipping from judicious deliberations into secular sermons. I awoke to these facts soon after I had joined the President's Council on Bioethics, when we began to discuss embryonic stem cells. The discovery of pluripotential, infi-nitely self-replicating stem cells early in the 1980s had lit up a whole domain of cellular and developmental biology and suggested thera-peutic approaches to chronic, debilitating, and incurable diseases such as Parkinson's and diabetes mellitus. But for some years, the U.S. government, knowing that harvesting the cells killed the em-bryos, would not fund research on stem cells that had been derived from human embryos.

On August 9, 2001, President George W. Bush made a thoughtful speech in which he proposed regulations permitting federal funding for research using stem-cell lines from human embryos that had been killed before that date. The National Institutes of Health, proceeding under this compromise, has since made fifteen to twenty human stem-cell lines available for federally supported research.

But as might have been expected, few serious participants in the debate were satisfied by this compromise. Most stem-cell specialists reject what they see as an arbitrary limit on their resources and programs—and, among other substantive objections, note that a boundary date for production eliminates the chance of improving the quality of stem cells (Gearhart, 2004). People who recognize a gift of individual human life in every embryo—an "end" in itself, not to be treated merely as a "means"—recoil at its destruction, no matter when or why it occurs. All of us on the President's Council on Bio-ethics—whose formation President Bush announced during that same August speech—developed our views on federal funding as we gathered information and exercised (vigorously, I can attest) our human talent for disagreement.

The concern that shadows the free use of human stem cells derives from disquiet over their origins. If a source other than embryos can provide pluripotential stem cells—and if harvesting them requires no killing—then this shadow vanishes. Thus, we all celebrate the discovery of stem cells in umbilical-cord blood, bone marrow, and other tissues.

But President Bush charged our council with thinking through the possibility of "cloning" as another source of human stem cells. This process, better termed somatic-cell nuclear transfer (SCNT), carries the potential of producing a living replica (clone) of the donor of a somatic-cell nucleus. It involves calling into play the genetic material and mechanisms that are latent in all somatic-cell nuclei, allowing them, under certain conditions, to recapitulate embryonic development and produce stem cells.

Ultimately, we council members were unanimous in many conclusions about cloning ("Human Cloning," 2002). We rejected the use of cloning for human reproduction. We agreed that regulatory measures should be developed for stem-cell cloning to guarantee, among other matters, that only qualified laboratories would receive federal support for work with human SCNT.

We were divided over whether research should be put on hold until the regulations are in place. A small majority (ten) of us favored a four-year moratorium on federal support to permit these regulations and oversight structures to be developed. A large minority (seven) of us believed that this work is so rich in therapeutic promise that it should proceed without delay and regulations could catch up with it.

It seemed to me that most of our disagreements rested on different attitudes generated, interestingly, by the same view of SCNT. This view maintains that there is no ethically important difference between a blastocyst derived from in vitro fertilization and one derived from SCNT. Thus, if one holds that deriving embryonic stem cells from in vitro fertilization should be illicit, this conclusion would also apply to SCNT, and vice versa.

I, however, see a distinction between the two procedures that sanctions different practices involving their products. In my view, SCNT resembles tissue culture, whereas in vitro fertilization represents instrumental support for human reproduction. Specifically,

SCNT is an engineered culturing of the nucleus of a somatic cell, accomplished by implanting this nucleus into an enucleated ovum, thereby forming a new diploid cell with the genetic characteristics of the "donor" of the nucleus. This new cell begins to replicate, following a developmental program that is latent in the genes of every somatic cell but which has been suppressed since it was employed in the original embryonic development of the donor organism.

I argue that this process of SCNT, by causing the expression of an intrinsic potential for growth and replication that is found in every somatic cell, can extend and expand a donor's cellular mass into extracorporeal space, as any form of tissue culture does. The stem cells that issued from the process would, in this view, be licitly used as the donor allowed. To specify this fundamental difference between in vitro fertilization and SCNT, I suggested that, since we call the first cell produced by fertilization the zygote, we dub the combination of nucleus and enucleated ovum that launches SCNT the "clonote."

Thus, I argue that in vitro fertilization entails the begetting of a new human being right from its start as a zygote and that we should use it to produce babies rather than cells or tissues to be harvested for purposes dictated by other human beings. In contrast, SCNT is a biologic manufacturing process that we may use to produce cells but should not use to produce babies.

My distinction rests on the origin of cells in SCNT, not on the process's vaunted potential for producing a living replica (clone) of the donor, as with Dolly the sheep. My confidence in making origins rather than potential the crux of the argument rests first on a reductio ad absurdum: if one used the notion of "potential" to protect cells developed through SCNT because with further manipulation they might become a living clone, then every somatic cell would deserve some protection because it has the potential to follow the same path. But I became more sure of this opinion when strong testimony was presented to the council (Jaenisch, 2003) indicating that SCNT performed with primate cells produces embryos with such severe epigenetic problems that they cannot survive to birth.

I still support the call of the council's small majority for SCNT regulations that will ensure, among other things, that human ova are not wasted like cheap reagents, or women pressed into service in unsafe ovum-production lines. Also, because I see that my argument supporting SCNT as a source of cells might easily justify growing the blastocysts to more advanced stages so as to harvest organs or tissues, I support limiting the existence of the clonote to fourteen days. When these regulations are in place, federal funding for biologic research on human stem cells derived through SCNT should proceed.

I continue to hold in principle—as do many Americans and governments of several Western nations—that using in vitro fertilization to generate harvestable cells and tissues represents a seriously problematic, life-disowning use of biologic science. But I also appreciate that practice with human embryonic stem cells has raced ahead of principle and that the president's compromise—restraining the practice but not banning research that could bring great benefits—was a wise one.

I'm asked what I would say if some other country's scientists, using methods unsupported in the United States, discovered a cure for parkinsonism, diabetes, or Huntington disease. But that's easy. First, I'd celebrate. I've not spent fifty years working and praying for such a victory to meet it without a welcome.

Then, after we'd drunk all the champagne, I'd surely ask, "What price this glory?" If we could reap the benefits using adult stem cells or SCNT, I'd lose no sleep over the methods that revealed them. If the therapies depended on trophic factors that we could extract and synthesize, I'd salute them. If the only effective therapies came with cells manufactured in factories where women were treated like battery hens, vats of sperm and ova bubbled and brewed, and human embryos were chopped and diced, I'd fret—as I fret over any product made under inhuman conditions.

But, even for bioethics, such matters lie too far in the future. The method I followed in arguing for SCNT remains compelling. Know the technical features through and through when working out the rightness or wrongness of a medical procedure. "God is in the details," noted the architect Ludwig Mies van der Rohe. Never has that truth echoed more loudly in the arena of biologic enterprise than it does now.

New England Journal of Medicine, 2004

REFERENCES

Gearhart, J. (2004). New human embryonic stem-cell lines—more is better. *New England Journal of Medicine* 350:1275–1276.
Human cloning and human dignity: The report of the President's Council on Bioethics. (2002). New York: Public Affairs.
Jaenisch, R. (2003). Testimony: President's Council on Bioethics, July 24, 2003. (Accessed June 22, 2004, at www.bioethics.gov/meetings.)

A Psychiatrist Looks at Terrorism

In the wake of September 11, what can a psychiatrist contribute to America's defense? Nothing, of course, to defend the nation from bombs, but something perhaps to defend it against confusion—and here America certainly needs help.

At the University of Pennsylvania, the provost called several neuroscientists together to consider whether the terrorists should be viewed as bad or mad: evildoers or sufferers from an exculpating mental disease. The group reached no conclusion, but one participant thought "brain images" might give the answer.

Editorialists argued about whether the atrocities should be considered acts of war or crimes. The blame-America-first group wanted the events called crimes and proposed prosecutions at The Hague. Some even opposed military retaliation, concerned that it would kill innocent people, produce martyrs, and generate recruits to the terrorist cause, along with endless war.

One distinguished Boston psychiatrist, speaking to anchorman Peter Jennings on ABC, explained the emotional distress of Americans as castration anxiety provoked by seeing the destruction of these two "phallic symbols" on the tip of Manhattan and suggested more psychoanalytic insight for us all.

Against this backdrop, there may be a place for some psychological realism—about what terrorists do, how they think, the steps necessary to protect ourselves from them, and the price those steps are likely to exact from us. The observations that follow spring from long clinical experience with similar matters. The citizen should judge them by the light of common sense and what he or she knows about the ways of the world. Where these insights overlap with and reinforce ideas from other relevant sources—diplomatic, legal, economic, military—they may enhance confidence in the course of action we must take.

A realist can begin by rejecting the castration-anxiety idea—even though it provided the only humor in the whole affair. Americans felt emotional distress not because the towers of the World Trade Center were longer than they were wide but because witnessing the cruel deaths of so many of our fellow citizens—horribly killed as they went about their daily lives, unsuspecting and unprotected—naturally provokes grief, anger, and fear. The brutal, indiscriminate slaughter of thousands of people in an instant, along with the sight of their bodies dropping like debris from dizzying heights, should produce pity, grief, rage in anyone with an ounce of fellow feeling.

Next, having rejected a far-fetched theory, the pragmatic behavioral scientist sets aside for the time being questions about whether the actions at issue were mad or bad, crimes or acts of war, and examines the phenomenon of terrorism itself. The hijacking of airplanes and the piloting of them as missiles into large buildings, he notes, the deliberate targeting of civilians with the aim of producing fear, dread, and their political profits, is purposeful action. It is behavior.

Terrorist behavior is different from behavior such as eating, drinking, or sex in that it springs not from any innate drive or instinctive motive but from a set of assumptions, attitudes, and beliefs that the actors have taken from their culture and share with many others. In contrast to their fellow citizens, however, these actors bring a ferocious passion to these ideas, a passion that leads them to ignore all other considerations such as personal safety, humane feelings, compromise, or temporizing alternatives.

In everyday speech, we call such people "fanatics." Psychiatrists, however, have their own, less loaded term. They say that people with this passionate attitude have an "overvalued idea." This conceptual distinction in mental life was first made by the late-nineteenth-century German psychiatrist Carl Wernicke.

An overvalued idea is a thought shared with others in a society or culture but in the patient held with an intense emotional commitment capable of provoking dominant behaviors in its service. An overvalued idea differs from a delusion in that delusions are false ideas unique to the possessor, whereas overvalued ideas develop from assumptions and beliefs shared by many others. An overvalued idea differs, too, from an obsession in that, although it dominates the mind as an obsession does, the subject does not fight an overvalued idea but instead relishes, amplifies, and defends it. Indeed, the idea fulminates in the mind of the subject, growing more dominant over time, more refined, and more resistant to challenge.

The major contemporary clinical disorder prompted by an over-valued idea is anorexia nervosa. Patients suffering from this illness take an idea common among young women in our society—thinner is better—and amplify it into a commitment so dominant that they starve themselves. At first an anorexic may claim that she is no different from any woman "thinking thin." As she persists with a worrisome starvation diet, she may justify eating only low-fat salads as her way to "health." All therapeutic attempts to correct the behavior by dissuading her of this idea or uncovering its root cause fail because the overvalued idea—one cannot be too thin—resists logical argument and compromise. Only stopping the behavior—which may require bringing the patient under twenty-four-hour supervision—can lead the anorexic to recover.

But overvalued ideas also crop up outside the clinical setting. Two recent examples of individuals with overvalued ideas are the Unabomber and Jack Kevorkian. The Unabomber, preoccupied with what he saw as the materialism and destructive reliance on technology of our society, carried out vicious and cowardly letter bomb assaults against many defenseless people he associated with these enterprises. When his rambling, expansive, and tedious explanations were published in the *Washington Post*, many readers reported that they agreed with much of what he said.

Jack Kevorkian, despite killing scores of sick, emotionally vulnerable people in Michigan, persuaded several juries that his ideas about assisted suicide were well intended, even though contrary to law. Juries repeatedly freed him, until his indiscriminate killing and disdain for the courts became too much to stomach. Kevorkian and the Unabomber now sit in jail because only incarceration could keep them from continuing their violence. Neither of them is mad in the sense of being out of contact with reality, but both of them are bad because of their vile opinions and vicious behavior. Their "brain images" would make no difference to such judgments.

Three historical figures with overvalued ideas are Adolf Hitler with his anti-Semitism, Carry Nation with her excessive devotion to temperance, and John Brown the abolitionist. Note that an overvalued idea may not in itself be wrong. Enough people agreed with Carry Nation to pass the Eighteenth Amendment; and all now agree with John Brown that slavery is evil, even though they deplore his assaults on defenseless farmers in Kansas and his killing spree at Harpers Ferry.

Overvalued ideas develop as ruling passions in some vulnerable individuals. Anorexics tend to be introverted young women, impressionable and easily conditioned by criticism of their physical appearance. The Unabomber, Jack Kevorkian, and the World Trade Center terrorists also tended to a personality type, arrogant and overconfident, suspicious of others, lacking in warmth, and tediously argumentative, shifting their ground to justify their fixed opinions when faced with strong objections. Cold, paranoid, and aggressive are terms that describe them. All efforts to correct the behavior of such people by addressing its "root causes" will fail because those "causes" are not actually motivating these people's behavior—their passions are.

Defining the September 11 attacks as behavior and the terrorists as men driven by the overvalued idea that America is a satanic nation whose citizens deserve death has implications for ways of defeating them. Here, recent psychiatric experience in treating behavior disorders can help.

Before about 1975, psychiatrists treating patients with destructive behaviors such as anorexia, alcoholism, and sexual disorders believed that one should first find the psychological roots of these behaviors by uncovering their meaning in the patient's mental conflicts. They thought that if these meaningful conflicts could be resolved, the abnormal behavior would wither away. This approach failed. Treatment programs for anorexia, for example, that ignored the failure to eat while attending to its meaning had death rates of between 10% and 15% of their patients. Alcoholics continued to drink, sex offenders to offend, even while their psychiatrists claimed to be reaching an understanding of their problems.

These results eventually caused doctors to try treatments that directly interrupted the harmful behavior. Anorexics were brought under dietary supervision, alcoholics were detoxified and sent to clinics implementing the twelve-step program of Alcoholics Anonymous, and sex offenders were given testosterone-suppressing medications and vigorous group therapy concentrated on discrediting their activities and their justifications. These treatments worked far better: many more anorexics, alcoholics, and sex offenders recovered.

This experience taught psychiatrists that behavior, once begun, maintains itself. Anorexics like to see their weight and dress size steadily shrink. Alcoholics, drug addicts, and sex offenders get immediate pleasurable reinforcement to continue their activities.

The same is true of terrorists: their behavior is maintained by its consequences, especially the publicity that draws attention to the terrorist and his or her ideas. The Unabomber hated to be pushed off center stage by Timothy McVeigh and so killed two more people right after the Oklahoma City bombing. Jack Kevorkian started videotaping his killings for CBS TV when Michigan ceased bringing him to court. Although the September 11 terrorists died in their assault, they were sure of worldwide publicity for their actions and their views. Their success brought dancing to the streets in certain Muslim cities and recruits to their war against America—far more recruits than any "root cause" of terrorism, such as poverty or anger at Israel, had brought.

By implication, then, to stop terrorism, the American government should devote its energies to interrupting the terrorists' behavior in all its aspects. The government should use every reasonable method to apprehend individuals who could carry out terrorist actions. It should protect vulnerable sites and situations. And most crucial, it should alter the consequences of the September 11 assault: to our injuries it should promptly add injuries to those responsible for the attack.

This policy should be judged simply and tough-mindedly by its success in preventing more terrorist behavior. Preventing terrorist events must be our prime aim, not just because each atrocity is an evil in itself but also because terrorism, like every other behavior, grows with its performance. To accommodate ourselves to it as a "fact of life" is to sustain it.

Our government can ignore certain matters for the moment. We should not expend much energy unearthing the "preconditions" for terrorism or pay credence to the justifying explanations offered by spokespeople for terrorists, no matter how reasonable they may seem. In truth, there are as many reasons offered for terrorism as there are terrorists—just as Alcoholics Anonymous has learned that there are as many reasons offered for drinking as there are drunks.

Stop the behavior first, and then, once peace is restored, we can deal with underlying issues. We will very likely find that many of the justifications now offered for terrorism were only rationalizations intended to excuse it. But we need not waste our energies trying to change the opinions of terrorists about us and our aims. These people, like the Unabomber and Jack Kevorkian, have overvalued ideas that are inaccessible to argument and persuasion. Their behavior will continue unless they are captured or killed.

Whether we call the terrorists' atrocities acts of war or crimes should be determined by one thing: which term best helps us stop the behavior. It seems more likely that we can keep terrorists from striking again if we treat them as soldiers captured committing acts of war on a battlefield of their own devising than if we treat them as individuals indicted for crimes and innocent until proven guilty. The IRA terrorists and sympathizers confined to the Maze prison at Long Kesh in Northern Ireland demanded the status of soldier-prisoners rather than criminal-prisoners. Certainly our laws can accommodate their Muslim counterparts.

Finally, what of the concern that military action will generate martyrs, draw recruits to the terrorists' cause, and produce endless conflict? Psychiatrists are familiar with this worry. It crops up whenever they propose a treatment aimed at interrupting a behavior. Patients and relatives all see and object to the intrusion on the patient's autonomy—such as the demand that the anorexic stay in a hospital so that her eating can be supervised or the requirement that the sex offender take libido-reducing medications. They wonder whether this will only cause patients to "dig in their heels" or "lose self-esteem." They propose that the psychiatrist should discover and resolve some meaningful conflict behind the behavior and so spare the patient a distressing treatment. Psychiatrists must explain to patients and their families that every effort to interrupt or change behavior elicits short-term losses, which are the price of recovery. Clinicians must weigh the inevitable short-term losses against the potential long-term gains.

Sometimes the likely losses are excessive. The classic illustration is stopping a lynch mob. One had best not attempt this alone, as the short-term cost to oneself could be terminal. Better to bring an army to stop a mob. Then, after order is restored and the hard feelings that are the short-term cost of preventing the crowd from working its will have dissipated, work to end the ideas and attitudes that support lynching.

In America's effort to interrupt the behavior of terrorists, many of whom are nestled in our country, the government may need laws that temporarily reduce civil liberties. We may have to go on a war footing, with special authority turned over temporarily to the military. We may have to sacrifice privileges in travel and tax relief. Discussion and careful judgments should aim to minimize and justify these losses. All such measures should be reassessed regularly. But they should be understood as the inevitable short-term costs of interrupting terrorist behavior.

The same sort of reasoning applies to our dealings with other countries. We have spent decades building up certain political and diplomatic relationships during peacetime. Some of these relationships will be damaged as we vigorously bring war to terrorists and their sympathizers and demand help from those who would call us friends. Again, we should consider what immediate losses might be irreparable and avoid actions that produce them. A nuclear winter would obviously be an unacceptable short-term cost. An increase in the vociferous complaining about America on Arab TV, however, can be expected and tolerated.

Some short-term costs deserve extensive discussion, informed by the concerns of diplomats, economists, lawyers, and others, before they are accepted or rejected. Psychiatrists have little to contribute to these proceedings other than to point out that the criterion for judging a policy is clear: if terrorist behavior continues, then—given that each successful attack makes subsequent attacks more likely—efforts to stop it should be enhanced, even though short-term losses will increase.

When we prevail in stopping terrorist behavior, we will likely discover much support for us in the oppressed Muslim world, support now hidden by the clamor for war. We can be sure that most Muslim mothers and fathers do not want their children lured to violent deaths in the name of some wild, overvalued idea promoted by charismatic tyrants whose own sons never get sent on suicide missions. Freedom will be welcomed once the majority can speak openly. We already see this in Afghanistan. The short-term losses of the bombing phase have been overcome by the joy of long-term release from the Taliban.

In sum, a realistic, pragmatic psychiatric depiction of terrorism— one that avoids dubious theories about meaning, as well as wishful thinking about how to manage it—can dispel confusion and offer a context for the understandings contributed by other disciplines. Thus, the proposals advanced here about managing terrorism fit with the idea of proceeding with a just war.

This approach allows us to assure our critics that, even as we know short-term losses to be inevitable when behavior must be changed, we also presume that many of the losses will be repaired by the long-term gains of success. All can agree that force and destruction are not enough for a sustained peace. Eventually we must repair some of what is damaged and develop our understanding of the grievances and concerns of our adversaries. To any who doubt our capacity to use more than force to gain a long-term peace, we can offer the historical instances of American magnanimity and devoted efforts at rebuilding where we had conquered, as after the Civil War and the two world wars of the twentieth century.

We are a forgiving people, but now, at the start of the first war of the twenty-first century, is the time for action—action directed by a coherent view of our adversaries and of what they are trying to do to us. Churchill defined these matters better than any psychiatrist. "Our aim," he said, "is victory, victory at all costs, victory in spite of all terror, victory, however long and hard the road may be; for without victory, there is no survival."

The Weekly Standard, 2001

CREDITS

"Annihilating Terri Schiavo." *Commentary* 119 (June 2005): 27–32. Reprinted by permission; all rights reserved.

"The Death of Freud and the Rebirth of Psychiatry." *The Weekly Standard* 5 (July 17, 2000): 31–36.

"Dissociative Disorder Is a Socially Constructed Artifact." *Journal of Practical Psychiatry and Behavioral Health* 1 (September 1995): 158–166.

"Dying Made Easy." *Commentary* 107 (February 1999): 13–17. Reprinted by permission; all rights reserved.

"The End of a Delusion: The Psychiatric Memory Wars Are Over." *The Weekly Standard* 8 (May 26, 2003): 31–34.

"Genius in a Time, Place, and Person." Foreword to Karl Jaspers, *General Psychopathology*, vols. 1 and 2 (Baltimore: Johns Hopkins University Press, 1997).

"Hippocrates à la mode." *Nature Medicine* 2 (May 1996): 507–509.

"How Psychiatry Lost Its Way." *Commentary* 108 (December 1999): 32–38. Reprinted by permission; all rights reserved.

"The Kevorkian Epidemic." *The American Scholar* 66 (Winter 1997): 15–27.

"No Veterinarian to 'The Naked Ape.'" *Cerebrum: The Dana Forum on Brain Science* 6, no. 4 (Fall 2004): 19–24. Copyright 2004 Dana Press, reprinted with permission.

"Psychiatric Misadventures." *The American Scholar* 61 (Autumn 1992): 497–510.

"A Psychiatrist Looks at Terrorism." *The Weekly Standard* 7 (December 10, 2001): 21–24.

"Psychiatry and Its Scientific Relatives: A Little More Than Kin and Less Than Kind." *Journal of Nervous and Mental Disease* 175 (October 1987): 579–583.

"Psychotherapy Awry." *The American Scholar* 63 (Winter 1994): 17–30.

"Romancing Depression." *Commentary* 112 (December 2001): 38–42. Reprinted by permission; all rights reserved.

"A Structure for Psychiatry at the Century's Turn: The View from Johns Hopkins." *Journal of the Royal Society of Medicine* 85 (August 1992): 483–487.

"Surgical Sex." *First Things* (November 2004): 34–38. Reprinted by permission.

"Treating the Mind as Well as the Brain." *The Chronicle of Higher Education* (November 22, 2002).

"What's the Story?" *The American Scholar* 64 (Spring 1995): 191–203.

"William Osler and the New Psychiatry." *Annals of Internal Medicine* 107 (December 1987): 914–918.

"Zygote and 'Clonote': The Ethical Use of Embryonic Stem Cells." *New England Journal of Medicine* 351 (July 15, 2004): 209–211. Copyright © 2004 Massachusetts Medical Society. All rights reserved.